T0003792

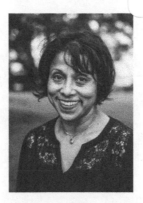

Himali McInnes is a family doctor who works in a busy Auckland practice and in the prison system. She writes short stories, essays, articles, flash fiction and poetry. She has been published locally and internationally. She was the inaugural Verb Wellington Writers Resident in October 2020. Her writing, whether fiction or non-fiction, often explores the theme of otherness. Himali is also a keen gardener, beekeeper and chicken farmer. She is obsessed with dogs and books.

The
unexpected
patient

The unexpected patient

Dr Himali McInnes

HarperCollinsPublishers

HarperCollins_Publishers_
Australia • Brazil • Canada • France • Germany • Holland • India
Italy • Japan • Mexico • New Zealand • Poland • Spain • Sweden
Switzerland • United Kingdom • United States of America

First published in 2021
by HarperCollins_Publishers_ (New Zealand) Limited
Unit D1, 63 Apollo Drive, Rosedale, Auckland 0632, New Zealand
harpercollins.co.nz

Copyright © Himali McInnes 2021

Himali McInnes asserts the moral right to be identified as the author of this work. This
work is copyright. All rights reserved. No part of this publication may be reproduced,
copied, scanned, stored in a retrieval system, recorded, or transmitted, in any form or by
any means, without the prior written permission of the publisher.

A catalogue record for this book is available from the National Library of New Zealand

ISBN 978 1 7755 4170 7 (pbk)
ISBN 978 1 7754 9201 6 (ebook)

Cover design by Darren Holt, HarperCollins Design Studio
Cover image by Chris Whitehead / Getty Images
Typeset in Adobe Garamond Pro by Kirby Jones
Author photograph by Alex Carter, One AM Creative

Ko te kaha kei te tinana, ko te mana kei te wairua.
The strength is in the body but the power is in the spirit.

CONTENTS

Introduction

For the last decade, I worked full-time as a GP. The rigours of general practice – the pivot shift to a new patient every 15 minutes, the holistic and relational long-term care, the gratitude of patients – are exhilarating. I utterly love being a GP. I also utterly love words. But full-time general practice meant that by the time I got home, I was leached of the mental energy needed to write. I'm definitely a morning person, and I probably photosynthesise for energy. I'm also an introvert. Post-work evenings saw me at a low ebb.

In mid-2019, I decided to work part-time in order to let word-bursts form at will. Then the Covid-19 pandemic happened, making 2020 a frightening and destabilising year for many. At no other time in history has both information and misinformation travelled so quickly. We collectively weighed the rights of the community versus the rights of the individual as we made choices over how we should act; meanwhile, the anxiety surrounding this virulent suckered pathogen glued us to our lit-blue screens for hours.

But with change can come unexpected opportunity.

By March 2020, as New Zealand's cases increased, general practice clinics reached a fever pitch of busyness. Colleagues fretted about the impending pandemic, about being on the front line with not enough protective gear. People stockpiled paracetamol and toilet paper. Then, as our strict lockdown was announced, general practice switched from traditional to mostly virtual consults. Clinics scrambled to set up telehealth services, and patients either contacted us from their homes or avoided bothering us altogether, concerned we'd be overrun with pandemic cases. Just like that, the swell of patients in our waiting rooms dwindled to a trickle. It was a peculiar chiaroscuro effect – the almost absurd opposite of normality.

At that time, Steve Braunias, silver-haired wizard of words, asked me to pen my thoughts on the effects of Covid-19 on general practice. For someone who reserves a particularly acerbic wit for the dotards of public life, Steve is also a kind and encouraging veteran to nascent writers like myself. Thanks to him, I wrote two essays for *Newsroom*, and then the idea for this book of medical stories emerged.

***

When I first graduated from the University of Auckland's School of Medicine, my head was full of facts, my hands scrambled to learn new skills and a fistful of fears anointed my daily practice. There was, for instance, the constant fear of making a mistake that might cost a life. Or of fainting onto the operating table while assisting a surgeon in theatre. Mostly, there was the anxiety of not performing to the expectations of senior colleagues. Being thrust into the thick of it during an overseas stint in the UK's NHS as a neonatal and paediatric registrar was hair-raising, but also fostered confidence. Once you've managed to get an intravenous (IV) line into a tiny hand, its skin as soft as butter; slipped an umbilical arterial catheter into a miniature abdomen; or aimed an endotracheal tube at a minuscule glottis and succeeded with its correct placement, you can't help but start to feel like a real doctor.

Although medical school was good at delineating the 'what' of medicine, it has taken me years of being at the coalface to appreciate the 'why'. I'm still learning. My focus has shifted from a solipsistic standpoint, with medic firmly at the centre, to become much more patient-centred (although there are days when I am too tired or busy to practise the sort of medicine that is truly holistic or fulfilling). Over time, and with the benefit of hundreds of patient interactions, I've started to think about the invisible things that push and pull at us. It's made me realise, time and again, that what I see on the surface of another human being is not the main thing, or the only thing. I try to keep this in mind with everyone I encounter; it is particularly pertinent during my shifts as a prison GP, where the patients' childhood stories are so vastly different from my own sheltered, cosseted childhood that I find it hard not to cry.

As my focus has shifted, I've noticed that it is not knowledge and skill alone which are important to patients. Instead, the sauce that begets richness is relationship. Kindness, compassion and appreciation of all the non-medical things that patients deem important and which leverage their health much more than pills.

Each medic–patient encounter described in *The Unexpected Patient* is profoundly affected by the unseen. By the things we carry: our beliefs, our experiences, our stories, our desires. By the patient's personality, but also by the life stories of their medical carers. I've long suspected that there is no such thing as a black-and-white diagnosis, or a perfectly dispassionate, factual and unemotional health professional. Our thoughts and feelings, our cognitive biases, do bleed into each consult, often without our conscious awareness.

***

There are 14 stories in total, which delve into each patient's case (with interviews from the patient themselves where possible), a little about the medic, and an exploration of a particular theme that each brings up. Every one of the patients has affected their health practitioner in unexpected ways, be it a nurse, doctor or trauma therapist. Some encounters were brief but powerful, and remained burnt into the medic's memory for years afterwards;

others did not seem that significant at the time, but became resonant with meaning later on.

Generational trauma and injustice affect people in enduring ways, not just economically but also through health, housing and even the function of our genetic code. This is at the heart of my own story of patient-triggered change. It's about a medic who was initially blind to the ills of colonisation, but who started to recognise the systemic issues that impacted her patient. My patient, after reading through 'their' chapter, sent me this note: 'Doc, thank you for listening to my story. You made it easier for me in letting go of other parts that I never thought possible.'

A paediatrician spoke of a midnight epiphany in which she recognised that the little Cambodian girl in front of her, a recurrent hospital attendee, was beset by multiple, clustered disadvantages. A retiring GP spoke of an obstetric patient's case, 40 years ago, which saw him tangled with hospital politics and an untenably busy workload. A surgeon, a familiar face from our television screens as New Zealand's first *Bachelorette*, spoke of a patient in denial who seemed to simply give up when confronted with her diagnosis. A South Auckland nurse remembered the woman who unexpectedly revealed a painful past, and what this revelation sparked in the nurse herself.

Another nurse spoke of the patient labelled a 'grump' by all the other staff, and how he informed her concept of culturally centred care. A Pākehā psychiatrist, whose ancestor a century ago was lauded by Māori for respectful partnership with them, spoke of his own work with a colleague that brought resolution and health for a Māori woman in a way that was sublimely tikanga Māori.

There's the fascinating story of a Canadian neurologist whose passion is metabolic medicine, and the Taupō-based patient who made it possible for him to express this passion more overtly. The deep south gave me the story of a personable, outgoing Geordie, and his incredible roadside rescue of a retired nurse on the brink of cardiac death. A rural GP reminisced about the patient who was almost a doppelgänger for himself, and of the unfairness that takes one young father but spares another. A straight-talking trauma therapist spoke of working inside a New Zealand prison, and the complexity of care and insight that is needed to understand the plight of prisoners. The Kiwi intensive care nurse who looked after the British prime minister when he was hospitalised with Covid-19 spoke of another patient who'd caused her to ponder the line between life and death, consciousness and unconsciousness.

In Wellington, a plucky prem baby, born at just 24 weeks, changed the practice of a neonatal nurse and the wider team looking after him. The Christchurch mosque attack victim I interviewed displayed such quiet courage, hope and resilience in the face of life-changing trauma that it wholly impressed his rehabilitation specialist.

Many interviewees, patient and medic alike, wished to remain anonymous. This is indicated at the start of each chapter with an asterisk next to their name. Others have given their real names. Patient details are in some instances altered for increased anonymity.

***

I've learnt so much writing these stories. They are a snapshot of the New Zealand health sector, and they span decades and specialties. They show us that our health, and the way we care for it, is influenced by so many things – from our past, our environment and our experiences to our lifestyles and what we ingest. Our health is even influenced by things that happened before we were born.

These stories remind us that what a patient deems most important may differ significantly from what their health practitioner deems most important. They are also a reminder to consider the unseen, to not make assumptions about others without fully understanding. Listening reaps dividends. Kindness begets kindness. It is not just health practitioners who give to their patients, but patients who give back to their health practitioners, in multiple tangible and intangible ways.

PART 1

Sudden events

PRIME time

patient: Carol*; clinical nurse specialist: Jony Lawson

It's one of the quintessential Kiwi dreams. To go travelling. To pare belongings down to the bare minimum, to grab a bag and go where the wind blows. No one to answer to, no particular place to be. But what happens when you are out and about in the 'wop-wops' and you suddenly become gravely ill, to the point of almost dying? How efficient is New Zealand's emergency rural health service?

***

Carol* has lived and worked in Dunedin her whole life. She started nursing at just 16 and for the next two decades worked at Dunedin Hospital, on the surgical ward mainly, and loved it. She did another decade in a retirement home, but then she tripped and fell, injured her right shoulder and had to have a year off work and lots of surgery. The MRI (magnetic resonance imaging) scan showed at least five torn muscles. When she'd healed enough to go back to work, multiple factors conspired against her. So, Carol decided to retire. After all, she was 65: she'd just received her Gold Card, her superannuation had kicked in, and she felt it was time to pursue some long-held dreams.

One of those dreams was to write a book about lighthouses, and to travel as she wrote. She sold her home in Dunedin and bought a motor home. It's spacious, has plenty of storage and is absurdly easy to drive – just like driving a car, she assures me. The only thing that's missing is a dog. When she left Dunedin, Carol left her beloved dog with her cleaner, who clearly also adored the animal. 'I'd love a big German Shepherd in the motor home with me,' says Carol. 'It'd be a good deterrent against some of the odd sorts you can meet while out on the road. But there'd be too much mess. It'd take too much time and energy to clean.'

Carol did a maiden voyage to Christchurch to see friends, and found that the freedom to go where she liked was liberating, fantastic. At the time of this story, she's on another road trip around the southernmost reaches of the South Island. However, Carol is unaware that she is about to experience a sudden severe medical emergency in the middle of nowhere.

***

It's January 2020. Earlier in the month, the skies had turned an eerie orange as the Aussie bushfires belched a fug of burnt eucalyptus into the skies above New Zealand. Carol is driving through the Catlins, and her friends are in convoy in another motor home as they all travel through this rugged area. It is a place of spectacular natural beauty. Carol is loving it – the space, the biting air. Inland, thick rainforests hug the hillsides voluptuously; to the north, the bush gives way to rolling farmland. The poet Hone Tuwhare lived in this area until his death, and his family plan to eventually set up a writer's retreat at his crib.

The convoy drives past sandy beaches washed in the cold brine of the Southern Ocean. Carol hopes to sight the rare, endangered yellow-eyed penguins, or at least the more common Hooker's sea lions and New Zealand fur seals. They stop to explore Nugget Point lighthouse – tentative research for her book.

As Carol and her friends sightsee, she's not her usual chirpy self. She feels out of sorts. The group watch the sea lions, then the others lope off on a short walk to stretch their legs but Carol opts to wait for them in her vehicle.

'I felt tired, fatigued, and I really didn't feel up to walking, which is not like me. But I didn't have any chest pain or anything at this stage.'

Carol's friends drive further down the coast. They're heading towards Invercargill to a dog show they want to attend. Carol turns left towards Curio Bay, with its historic petrified forest. There's a small settlement called Niagara en route to the bay and she stops for lunch at the Niagara Falls Cafe, enjoys a blue cod burger and chips.

'That's when I started to get the pain. It was a dull pain, like an elephant sitting on my chest. I thought, "Here we go, it's my indigestion again." I'd had similar pains before. However, this time it was much worse.'

Carol keeps driving. She now feels hot and clammy. She starts to wonder if this pain is actually something more sinister. A heart attack, even. She's got risk factors for this – her grandfather died of a heart attack at 65. Carol's father was an avid tramper, and fit, but he had a turn while out in the wilderness one day and had to slow to a dawdle. When he was investigated, there was an 80-per cent blockage in one of his coronary arteries. Carol herself is a Type II diabetic, and not a particularly well-controlled one. She says she is unable to tolerate many medications, and is more of a fervent believer in the importance of nutrition as treatment. Despite this family history and her diabetes, Carol pushes the thought that her chest pain might be a heart attack to the back of her mind.

'I didn't feel short of breath. I didn't have that feeling of doom. So I sort of convinced myself that it was just indigestion.'

As she drives through Tokanui, she sees the rural health clinic beside the road and thinks about stopping to get some help but there's no place to park her motor home. Ten minutes later, at Fortrose, she comes across a cemetery and an adjacent gorse-riddled paddock with plenty of parking. A farmer's house is nearby. Carol pulls off the road. Her chest pain is not going away. She stumbles out of her vehicle and drags herself over to the farmhouse, slowly, struggling for breath.

'I knocked on the door,' Carol says. 'When the farmer answered, I said to him, "Mate, can you call an ambulance? I'm not feeling too well. I think I've got indigestion."'

Carol sits down on the old wooden steps. The porch, with its commanding view over the fields, is a jumble of Red Band gumboots, rusty equipment and a sofa with unspooling stuffing. The farmer calls the nearest health centre – the one 13 kilometres away that Carol passed on her way here. Rural nurse Jony Lawson answers. It's 1.15 pm.

The farmer tells Jony, 'A lady's just come in off the road. She's had a dodgy pie. Says she's got indigestion and wants the ambulance, eh.' The farmer gives Carol some indigestion tablets, which do not help.

***

Jony arrives in a flurry of gravel in his emergency-response truck, a RAV4 kitted out with medications. Jony is a clinical nurse specialist, employed by the Southern District Health Board (DHB) to cover on-call shifts for PRIME, the Primary Response in Medical Emergencies service. This is a network of general practitioners and nurses trained to respond to emergencies in rural areas, especially where the ambulance service may take too long or where extra medical skills are required. Jony is also a certified flight nurse, having trained with the Royal Flying Doctor Service in Australia. Carol is in very good hands.

'I took one look at this lady, and I immediately thought, she's having an MI [myocardial infarction],' says Jony. 'Carol looked terrified. She was sweaty and grey, clutching her chest, said her pain was ten out of ten. The pain wasn't radiating to her neck or arm, but she did feel nauseous. I asked the farmer to call 111.'

This puts a call to St John so they can respond with an ambulance and possibly a helicopter. Jony gives Carol 300 mg of aspirin and some glyceryl trinitrate (GTN) spray under her tongue. This is a quick-acting medication that helps dilate blood vessels throughout the body. In an acute heart attack, where blood flow to the heart muscle is compromised by blockages, GTN can bring immediate relief. But for Carol, it has no effect.

Jony wants Carol to come inside so that she can lie down, but she says, 'No, I'm happy sitting here on the steps, thanks.' She's actually not sure if she'll be able to walk inside. She's too scared to move. The ambulance driver arrives, in another flurry of gravel. Carol is now persuaded to go into the ambulance to lie down. The town paramedic arrives 15 minutes later.

Jony places some defibrillator pads on Carol's chest to check her heart rhythm. This shows she's not in ventricular tachycardia – a dangerous rhythm that can lead to cardiac death, and which often requires treatment with a jolt of electrical cardioversion to shock the heart back to a normal rhythm. She's in a regular sinus rhythm instead, but Jony can see obvious ST-segment elevation on the rhythm strip. This abnormality of the electrical conduction of the heart indicates heart-muscle damage. He informs the comms team that he's dealing with a 'code red cardiac'.

Next, Jony does a 12-lead ECG (electrocardiogram: a recording of the electrical activity of the heart). This confirms an anterior STEMI. A STEMI is a ST-segment elevation myocardial infarction – a heart attack with particular changes on the ECG. Cardiologists have a mantra: 'Time is muscle.' The longer an MI is left untreated, the more heart-muscle damage occurs, and the greater the risk of dangerous arrhythmias and/or death.

With the confirmation and support of the town paramedic, Jony activates a 'code STEMI', using an app on his phone to alert the St John clinical desk. The air desk is also alerted, a helicopter is dispatched and Dunedin Hospital's cardiology staff are alerted. The app also has protocols for a variety of other conditions: stroke, atrial fibrillation (where the top chamber of the heart writhes in a chaotic fashion like a bag of worms), bradycardia (a slow heart rate), and cardiogenic shock (low heart output due to intrinsic cardiac causes).

Jony works through the STEMI checklist, which gives drug doses tailored to the patient's weight, timing of administration and so on. Two other intensive care paramedics, manning the clinical desk, work through the checklist at the same time as the ECG is sent electronically to them. 'As she's legally my patient, I do all the drugs, and with each one we carefully check off the thrombolysis checklist,' says Jony. 'I can do a wee bit more drugs-wise than the paramedic so it's a good team.'

What will save Carol's life is thrombolysis: medication that will work to rapidly dissolve the blood clot in her coronary arteries. Nowadays, many St John intensive care paramedics carry thrombolysis kits. They can be used for patients with myocardial infarctions or many cases of stroke; the underlying pathology in both is a blood clot that needs to be dissolved to allow blood flow to be restored.

***

Before March 2019, thrombolysis in New Zealand could only be activated within a hospital setting. PRIME responders with thrombolysis kits are a relatively recent development. Although it's a big deal, and the potential for causing more damage is omnipresent, it saves lives, especially in remote areas where patients can be hours from the nearest hospital.

'There's lots of contraindications to thrombolysis,' says Jony. 'I'm very careful. I probably overthink it a bit. I often ring the St John clinical desk – there's one in Christchurch, Dunedin and Auckland – for advice on clinical problems. If I can't get through to the clinical desk, I sometimes ring ED [emergency department].'

Any contraindications are reviewed by everyone involved. As the thrombolytic medication will target not only the coronary artery clot but the whole body, bleeding is a significant side effect. So, anyone with surgery, trauma or brain injury in the last six weeks cannot have it. Anyone who's had an ischaemic stroke in the last six months or an intracerebral haemorrhage (bleed in the brain) cannot have it. If a patient has had more than ten minutes of CPR (cardiopulmonary resuscitation) they should only be cautiously offered thrombolysis. It's a tight protocol.

Jony has helped to thrombolyse patients before, but always in the relatively controlled environs of a hospital and as part of a large team. Thrombolysing someone in a roadside emergency is on a whole new level. The potential for error is high. He feels a little nervous, but remains focused, thorough and works as quickly as possible.

Carol's oxygen saturations are now 95 per cent on 3 litres of oxygen. Her blood pressure is 199/100. This will need to be brought down before she can be thrombolysed. Jony gives her more GTN. Carol also needs intravenous access so she can get morphine for her pain. 'But I'm very demanding,' she says. 'I know that when patients get an IV line in the crook of their arm, it's a real hassle. So I said to Jony, "No, you're not allowed to put the line in my elbow or my left hand, but you can use my right hand."'

Jony manages to get the line in. He gives Carol 2 mg of morphine in increments, up to a total of 10 mg, over ten minutes, with little effect. Fentanyl, in 20-mcg increments, is given for the pain. Jony now administers a cocktail of thrombolysis medications: 300 mg clopidogrel orally, 50 mg IV of tenecteplase, 100 mg clexane into the skin of Carol's stomach, 5000 units of heparin via a slow infusion 15 minutes after the tenecteplase. Carol's blood vessels are now coursing with drugs. Because her blood pressure remains high at 200/100, Jony gives her 2 mg metoprolol through the IV line as well. He measures her blood pressure, heart rate and perfusion every ten minutes. He does another ECG, which shows that the ST changes are resolving.

The local fire service arrives and clears a space in a nearby paddock for the helicopter to land, and by the time it whizzes in 40 minutes later, Carol's pain is down to almost zero. She gives her keys to the farmer; her friends will pick up her motor home later. She's never been in a helicopter before. 'Unfortunately the paramedics made me lie down so I couldn't see a thing! It wasn't that much fun in the end. Plus, I was feeling nauseous.'

Once she lands at Dunedin Hospital, she is taken straight to the cardiac catheterisation laboratory. A stent is inserted into her blocked coronary artery to keep it patent. In all, it's taken less than 150 minutes from the first responder callout to Carol getting catheterised.

After the procedure, she feels great – virtually back to normal. She calls her daughter in Perth at half past three that same afternoon. 'Hi, darling, don't panic, I'm all right, but I've just had a heart attack.'

Looking back, Carol is in awe at how her life was saved. From Jony, to the helicopter, to the cath lab, it was such a smooth operation.

***

Jony Lawson was born in Durham, north-east England. Growing up, he wanted to be a famous footballer, or a troubadour touring the world. He was 'quite naughty' as a boy. 'I was too interested in the outside world to pay attention in class. I kept getting into trouble. Nonetheless, I got A grades in politics, so they persuaded me to go to uni to study politics.'

He was 18, and he lasted just 18 months before dropping out. 'No one should go to university that young. I should have just waited until I was 25 or something.' Jony took a year off and worked as a healthcare assistant. His sister, who is a mental-health nurse, persuaded him to give nursing a go, so he trained in Newcastle and Glasgow. 'She told me that nursing is not that difficult. Actually, it's not that easy! I was the least-likely nurse. The main things I guess were that I liked people a lot and I had an inquisitive mind.'

He worked in intensive care (ICU) and loved the autonomy of it, the adrenaline, the life-and-death scenarios. Transporting patients on flights also appealed for the same reasons. Then he met 'the love of his life' during a visit to Melbourne, and followed her back to New Zealand. They had a son, but the relationship itself didn't work out. Meanwhile, Jony passed the Royal Flying Doctor course in Australia and was asked to set up a flight-nurse service in the Bay of Plenty and Waikato.

'I worked for Philips Search & Rescue Trust (PSRT). I also helped set up the autonomous flight-nurse role, while I still was in ICU. I worked on the chopper and fixed wing for approximately ten years, which I *loved* – the only reason I left is because they controversially centralised the service.'

Jony moved to his current position at Tokanui 15 months ago. He does five days a week, with eight official hours on, but is on call 24 hours a day for PRIME (any 111 calls in the area that require him get directed through to his pager). Sometimes the on-call shifts are quiet. Other times, they're tremendously busy. He's only stood himself down once from search and rescue in eight years, after a particularly busy shift on the Rotorua air ambulance when he was so tired he could barely think. But at Tokanui, there is no one to replace him at short notice, and so he has to manage tiredness, illness and time off wisely. Jony does shifts on Stewart Island/Rakiura also.

'Sometimes with autonomous jobs you can end up being a bit gung-ho, but I take my clinical autonomy very seriously. It's great having backup. I always try and follow up my patients afterwards.'

When he's not working, he's enjoying the desolate southern beaches, the space, the fresh air. 'The area I cover for PRIME is large and remote, but also incredibly beautiful. I love it.'

Jony says he's grateful for the medical system in New Zealand. 'A year and a half ago, I did a stint of work in the Caribbean. The medical system there is aligned with the US. If patients need airlifting, they have to cough up the flight bill upfront. Up to 30,000 US dollars! If they can't afford to pay, and let's face it, how many people have a spare 30,000 bucks lying around, they have to wait for the next available commercial flight instead.

Whereas here in New Zealand, if anything goes wrong, you can almost always be fixed, and often without paying a penny.'

***

How can a patient such as Carol, a diabetic with a family history of heart disease, have had such a good outcome, despite being so far from a hospital?

PRIME, administered by St John, augments what is provided by the rural ambulance service both in speed of response and level of clinical expertise. In areas such as the Catlins, an ambulance might only be staffed by non-medical volunteers trained in first aid. Although New Zealand is not a large country, there are many scenarios in which time is a crucial commodity, as in Carol's case.

Rural medicine can be challenging. Populations are small and widely dispersed, and terrain can be rugged, making access difficult. Until the early 1990s, rural GPs coordinated with their local emergency services. Then, everything became centralised. The ambulance, fire and police first responders reported back to their respective headquarters; coordination disintegrated. In 1994, there was a public outcry following unsatisfactory emergency responses at two accidents in the South Island.

Retired GP and one of the founders of PRIME, Dr Trevor Walker, helped to spearhead the development of this new integrated service. 'I took three months off and toured the length of the South Island. I met loads of people in various towns, all the emergency first responders I could get hold of. I collected information and helped formulate the next steps.'

A number of issues were noted. Ambulance services were fragmented, acute health agencies used different protocols and guidelines, and networking and coordinating were inadequate. Patients were sometimes sent to the nearest hospital rather than the one that could provide the best care for their illness or injury. This wasted potentially life-saving time.

It was Trevor Walker who coined the term PRIME. The aim was to put together a national pre-hospital acute management system. Rural GPs needed to be part of the mix, air and land ambulance services needed to be integrated, and regional hubs in one of the five tertiary centres needed to coordinate local emergency care. The PRIME service got underway in the South Island in 1998, and in the North Island two years later. Nowadays, PRIME is administered and coordinated by St John, using funds provided by the Ministry of Health (MoH) and the Accident Compensation Corporation (ACC).

When a call for medical help is received, whether through the 111 service or via a non-urgent line, it is triaged by the local Ambulance Clinical Control centre. To mobilise a PRIME responder, the situation must be either immediately life-threatening or potentially life-threatening, and the location of the incident must be 30 or more minutes from the closest available paramedic ambulance. Carol's case fitted both criteria.

Currently there are 76 PRIME sites in New Zealand, from Stewart Island/Rakiura, east to Rēkohu/Chatham Islands, and up to Great Barrier Island and the Far North of the North Island. There are about 660 responders – about 60 per cent are nurses, 40 per cent doctors. From July 2019 to June 2020, they responded to about 2800 medical and accident-related calls around the country.

'The most fundamental thing you learn during the PRIME training course is the importance of teamwork,' says Dr Janette Bills, who is also Walker's partner and has been a member of PRIME since its inception. 'You find out ways to cut people out of vehicles. You learn how to defibrillate, do cardioversion, pace someone's heart. In the old days, we'd intubate and put people on portable ventilators. You learn how to insert an interosseous line into someone's tibia for IV access. These days, using a drill makes it so much easier in adults; however, practitioners have to buy the drill themselves as it's not yet in the PRIME kits.'

There are downsides to the PRIME service, and a major issue is funding. 'We used to basically do our on-call shifts for free. If we didn't get called out, we didn't get paid for the hours we were on call,' says Bills. 'Even today, being a member of PRIME can be a disadvantage to a practice, as it ends up subsidising the service at least some of the time. Some practices have responded by deciding not to provide after-hours care. This means that some areas don't have adequate emergency cover. Nowadays, people do want to be reimbursed for the time they work – which seems eminently fair!'

ACC will fund injuries, but about three-quarters of PRIME callouts are medical emergencies. These can take hours, and use up multiple consumables. PRIME sites receive some funding from MoH for these callouts, but this funding has been widely acknowledged as inadequate. The New Zealand Rural General Practice Network and other stakeholders are currently reviewing funding for emergency medical and trauma callouts.

There is also an emotional toll to being a PRIME responder. Frequently, they will be called to an emergency to find that the patient they are attending to is a neighbour or friend or relative. Janette Bills recalls the horrifying death of a young child on a farm, where a father had accidentally run over his son with a tractor.

'I thought I coped okay at the time. But when I got home, my little girl came running towards me with a bump on her head, and I broke down,' Bills recalls. 'I was just a young mum myself at the time. I couldn't sleep for weeks afterwards.' Nowadays PRIME responders have access to the St John peer-support team for a debrief, or they can access the counselling service.

Many rural GPs are nearing retirement and it is hard to find permanent replacements. The locums who fill in often do not have the same level of emergency-response experience. Thus rural nurses, including nurse specialists such as Jony, are a vital component.

'It's amazing that our nurses step up and take on a lot of the workload, including PRIME callouts,' says Bills. 'Rural nurses are an exceptional bunch. They are absolutely the backbone of rural health.'

As Carol cruises along New Zealand roads following her lighthouses, she could not agree more.

A benediction from beyond

patient: Mario*; intensive care nurse: Jenny McGee

There's no particular trick to looking after a prime minister. No particular sleight of medical hand that is needed, no singular zeal, no extra attention or special treatment. Just competent medical care. Methodical, thorough, relational. The sort of work that intensive care nurse Jenny McGee is excellent at and does during every shift, for every one of her patients.

In April 2020, UK Prime Minister Boris Johnson is admitted to St Thomas' Hospital after he falls ill with Covid-19. His jaunty shock of platinum-blond hair looks subdued in the Twitter message he posts just prior to being admitted. Initially, he is put on oxygen as a 'precautionary measure'. When he is moved into ICU, the possibility of mechanical ventilation, coma and potential death hovers. A head of state dying of illness during a pandemic is a frightening, destabilising proposition for many reasons.

After Johnson improves and is released, he credits 'Jenny from New Zealand' and nurse Luis Pitarma from Portugal for the exemplary care he received, saying that while his life hung in the balance, these two nurses kept vigil by his bedside and helped him to pull through.

Jenny is taken aback by the media fanfare that ensues. She just wants to get on and do what she is trained to do. To slip back into anonymity again. However, she handles herself with aplomb, with that practical get-on-with-it attitude that the prime minister so admired. She is interviewed on the news, and is calm and professional throughout, managing to inform viewers of facts in a way that is neither salacious nor breaches the PM's privacy. She is invited to high tea at Downing Street, alongside other team members who helped in his care. Jenny does laugh ruefully, though, that Invercargill 'gets all the glory' as her home town, after Johnson talks about this to the media. 'I actually grew up about 40 minutes out of Invercargill in a place called Edendale!'

Jenny has looked after many patients in ICU. Despite the worldwide scrutiny over the British prime minister's admission, it's another patient, called Mario*, who Jenny really finds hard to forget. Despite being comatose, this patient startled her with an apparent message for his grieving family.

***

Mario, a man in his sixties, ends up in the intensive care unit after surgery to remove necrotic bowel. He has a history of high cholesterol, and in the same way that fatty deposits can narrow heart arteries (in a process known as atherosclerosis), the arteries supplying blood to the small and large intestines can be similarly narrowed. This gives Mario intestinal angina for some years: abdominal cramping after eating that lasts one to three hours, low-grade abdominal pain, bloating and nausea. Mario controls his atherosclerosis well enough by modulating his blood pressure and taking a cholesterol-lowering medication known as a statin.

But one day he feels unwell. His heart rate feels odd, fluttery, like a small frightened bird skittering in his chest. Then he is hit with intense abdominal pain around his belly button that does not go away. He develops loose, slightly bloody stools, he becomes bloated and uncomfortable. He tries to wait it out for a few hours, hoping things will improve by themselves. But they don't. His worried family rush him to hospital.

The medical staff assess Mario and find that his heart is in atrial fibrillation, a relatively common irregular rhythm in those over 65 years of age. The two top chambers of his heart are not contracting normally because of chaotic electrical signals. This inefficient heart action causes low blood pressure, which in turn leads to poor blood supply to vital organs. Atrial fibrillation can also create blood clots. It is possible that a clot has become lodged in Mario's gut arteries. The already narrowed arteries, combined with the sudden further drop in blood flow, has likely caused his gut to become ischaemic (lacking in blood supply) and then necrotic (cells prematurely dying).

When Mario is admitted, his abdomen is bloated and tender. He looks pale and sweaty. He has a fever, a fast heart rate, low blood pressure, and is thought to have sepsis. An urgent CT scan shows pneumatosis intestinalis – gas within the wall of the bowel. This confirms that parts of his bowel are severely affected and are already dying or dead. Mario is rushed to theatre for surgeons to perform an emergency exploratory laparotomy.

They make a large vertical cut down his midline, from just below his xiphisternum (the pointy bone at the end of the breastbone) almost to his groin. They suction out blood-streaked watery fluid around his internal organs. Sections of his bowel are lifted out and examined methodically: from the duodenum, the first part of the small intestine, through to the rectum. Some sections of small bowel – about 70 centimetres of jejunum – have the dusky discolouration of ischaemia. Some sections are so dark they look like blood sausage. Staples are inserted to demarcate healthy gut from ischaemic gut. The nonviable sections are removed, and the abdomen is left open as part of a laparostomy.

The intention is to examine Mario later, intra-operatively, to see if further gut has died and needs resecting. Unfortunately, he suffers a cardiac arrest in theatre. Although his heart is brought back into a viable rhythm, the period of reduced blood flow to his brain sets the stage for later events.

***

Mario is moved to ICU, where Jenny and her team take over. He is sedated for comfort, intubated, given intravenous pain relief (a fentanyl infusion) and fluids. He is in a medically induced coma. Broad-spectrum antibiotics wash through his system to try to fight the sepsis that has seeded from his damaged gut to the rest of his body. A nasogastric tube runs from his nose to his stomach and drains off gastric fluid to prevent regurgitation into his lungs. His electrolyte and fluid status are monitored carefully. He receives nutrition intravenously, to allow his gut to rest. However, it becomes apparent that the surgery has occurred too late to be successful. Toxins from Mario's intestines, normally sealed within the gut, have leaked through the damaged gut walls and into his bloodstream.

Normally, our gut cells provide our first line of defence against invasion by potential pathogens. We have a lot of bacteria and viruses in our gut; someone who weighs 70 kilograms may have 100 trillion microbes in their gut (the combined weight of a fleshy mango). A person with a rich, varied gut microbiome appears to have a healthier immune system, and may be less liable to develop diseases of chronic inflammation such as diabetes, dementia and atherosclerosis. A poor variety of gut microbiota, conversely, has been linked to obesity.

When our little microscopic gut pets are fed properly (preferably with a plant-based diet that is varied and rich in fibre), they hum with pleasure, and this has manifold benefits. Microbes

31

produce essential short-chain fatty acids, via fibre breakdown, vital for healthy cell function in our bodies. They facilitate the absorption of important minerals such as magnesium, calcium and iron. They synthesise important vitamins such as vitamin K and folate, as well as create amino acids (the building blocks of proteins). Lastly, they produce the mood chemicals serotonin and dopamine. Researchers have found that those with a higher quality of mental health show a propensity to certain beneficial gut bacteria.

Our gut microbes can be adversely affected by antibiotics. These drugs are incredibly useful, but only when used appropriately for bacterial infections (*not* viral infections), as each time we have a course of these drugs, our gut bacteria can be depleted for several months. A diet scarce in fibre and plants can severely restrict the function and diversity of our gut bugs.

The lining of our intestines has a well-developed system of highly specialised epithelial cells with tight connections, mucus and immune cells to keep our gut microbiota inside our guts. In the right space, in the right place. When this integrity is damaged, as it is in Mario's gut because of the acute-on-chronic interruption to blood flow, leading to lack of oxygen and cell death, the intestinal cells swell with fluid and then rupture. Bacteria invade the dead cells, multiply, and create toxins and breakdown products that leak into the circulation. As these toxins circulate, they trigger immune-system hyperdrive. They also lead to multi-organ failure. It is very difficult to treat or reverse this cascade once in motion.

***

One by one, Mario's organs start to fail. First to succumb are his liver and kidneys; these soft, fleshy organs are particularly susceptible to toxic shock. He develops paralytic ileus in his gut, acute respiratory distress syndrome in his lungs, and impaired blood flow to his heart and brain.

The ICU consultant considers Mario's worsening clinical situation. She knows that the mortality rate is almost 100 per cent for patients with necrotic ischaemic gut with widespread sepsis, even with early recognition, resuscitation and surgical intervention. Mario's numbers are looking increasingly grim, with rocketing kidney and liver impairment, unstable blood pressure and an ongoing need for mechanical ventilation. His body has become acidotic (normal human arterial pH lies between 7.35 and 7.45; acidity below a pH of 6.8 can become incompatible with life).

Neurological tests to assess his brain function reveal that Mario is in a state of profound unresponsiveness due to the hypoxic (lack of oxygen) injury to his brain, sustained during the earlier cardiac arrest. He cannot open his eyes or speak, he is dependent on his ventilator, and he cannot exhibit purposeful behaviours. His body has lost its normal sleep–wake cycles. His brainstem shows depressed function, as evidenced by the failure of his pupils to react to light.

He is almost certainly progressing towards brain death: the irreversible cessation of all functions of the entire brain, including the brainstem. Once this occurs, there is no chance of revival. The difficult topic of palliation is broached with the family. This will involve removing Mario's breathing tube and keeping him as comfortable as possible while nature takes its course. Ultimately, the decision to palliate rests with the ICU consultant, not with the family. However, nothing is done without a family's express support.

'Sometimes, relatives oppose our decision to palliate,' says Jenny. 'But rarely do we need to enforce judicial authority to do what we think is medically best. At the end of the day, patients will declare themselves, sooner or later. For example, they may progress to cardiac arrest, but this can be undignified and traumatic for the family, especially if they then insist on CPR. We far prefer to palliate patients. It is more dignified and allows time for family to arrive. It's important to let relatives come to this understanding themselves.'

Mario's family are resistant to the idea that the medical staff be allowed to 'control' Mario's death. They are Orthodox Christians; to them, interfering is tantamount to playing God. Instead, they cluster around his bedside. They hold his hands, they weep, they implore him to give them a sign as to whether he is happy for treatment to be stopped. Jenny and her colleagues are sure that Mario will not be able to give the family the sign they desperately want. The patient has been unresponsive for days at this stage. He has not opened his eyes, breathed on his own or shown any purposeful movements.

Jenny has never forgotten what happens next.

Mario's eyes flutter open. He looks up to the ceiling. He raises his right hand upwards, wrist bent backwards, palm facing his family. It looks like a benediction. It looks like he is pointing towards the heavens. He then closes his eyes and is still. This is undoubtedly the sign the family members have been waiting for. They interpret it as Mario telling them that it's okay, that he's ready to move on. The tension around the bed dissolves. They hug each other. They are more at peace, and give the ICU team the go-ahead to palliate Mario.

**

Jenny McGee grew up on a farm, in the region known somewhat prosaically as Southland. She was obsessed with animals, and wanted to be a vet or a horse trainer when she grew up. After her older brothers went travelling, Jenny decided to become a nurse in order to work overseas and travel at the same time. 'I'm hugely social. I love seeing different cultures and learning new things,' she says.

She trained in New Zealand, then headed to Australia. A nursing friend persuaded her to try ICU, and she fell in love with it. 'I love the acuity of ICU, the in-your-face nature of it. The life-and-death issues. I thrive on that level of stress. I think I cope well because I'm organised and methodical and I just adapt to things. I also love the technology and science of ICU. The autonomy of the nurses is a big plus.'

Jenny next travelled to the UK and started work in the NHS. She's been there for ten years now. She thinks the NHS staff do a fantastic job. As an ICU nurse, she says she has 'open views' about life and death. 'If a family wants to do something unusual for a loved one, then I'm all for it. Why not? If it helps them grieve better, then it's a good thing. There are no rules.'

The process of some ICU patients dying has been accompanied by pet dogs or loud rock music. Families vividly remember how their loved ones died. Jenny and her ICU colleagues receive letters all the time thanking them for allowing people to have a dignified death. One patient really wanted to die at home. Jenny was charge nurse that day and says it was a race against the clock. The ambulance staff were reluctant to transport such an unstable patient. The patient was hard to mobilise as there was so much medical paraphernalia that needed to be moved alongside him. Jenny was exhausted afterwards. 'But it was worthwhile. He made it home. He ate a banana, then he died an hour later. We got a lovely email from his family thanking us profusely.'

In Mario's case, he was in an open ward with 12 other patients and only a curtain for privacy. He was too unwell, too unstable to move into a side room. His family were by his bedside: his two daughters, his son, his son's wife. As the days passed, their initial hopes that Mario would improve, that he would open his eyes, started to fade. The family's grief was public and remonstrative, with wailing and loud crying.

'People respond to grief so differently,' says Jenny. 'Some cultures, such as those from the Mediterranean, are very vocal and expressive. In British or Kiwi families – and this is a big stereotype, but there's some truth to it – there's more of a stiff-upper-lip thing. Grief is more private. There are probably some advantages to public or at least communal grief, I think.'

***

In order for us to maintain consciousness, we need intact function in the grey matter of both cerebral hemispheres (the wrinkled, walnut-like outer surface on the two halves of the brain) and also a working reticular activating system (RAS). The RAS is an extensive network of fibres and cells running through our brainstems and up through our midbrains. It helps regulate arousal and the stages of sleep. To impair consciousness, either both of our cerebral hemispheres, or the RAS, must be affected; a one-sided cerebral hemisphere injury only rarely causes unconsciousness.

Consciousness is not an on/off entity. Rather, it is a bit like sliding into deep water. The deeper you go, the less you are aware of what's happening on the surface. W. H. Auden's 'The Labyrinth' captures this enigmatic state:

The centre that I cannot find
Is known to my Unconscious Mind;
I have no reason to despair
Because I am already there.

Consciousness is an extraordinarily varied state and sometimes we may cycle between different levels of it. It requires both wakefulness and awareness. Wakefulness, a quantitative measure of consciousness, is having the ability to open your eyes and to display basic reflexes such as the cough or swallow reflex.

Awareness, on the other hand, is generally associated with complex thought processes and is consequently more difficult to assess. It's more of a qualitative measure, with fluid parameters such as attention, language, time and space orientation, and the ability to judge reality. It includes awareness of the self, of bodily signals, of thoughts, of the environment. Medics use proxy physical responses during an examination to detect awareness, and to detect the function of the cerebral cortices and the brainstem.

Of course, even while we are fully awake, many things can be outside our conscious awareness. Take the proverbial noisy party. With so much noise and chit-chat, we tend to focus on the person in front of us, yet some part of us is aware of our surroundings because we'll prick our ears up if our name or an interesting topic is mentioned across the room.

Sleep is a unique state of consciousness where we have partial awareness and where the brain is still active. The boundary between waking from sleep and full wakefulness is fluid; some teenagers, for example, may appear to be awake when they are dragged from their beds and made to go to school, but in fact may not possess full awareness of their surroundings until many hours later. Some stages of sleep are more of a conscious state than other stages, especially REM sleep when we are dreaming. Deep non-REM sleep could more correctly be labelled a state of unconsciousness. Dr Matthew Walker, in his book, *Why We Sleep*, postulates that REM sleep is akin to a form of psychosis. The full reality of sleep may be a web of fluidity, an alchemy of heterogenous states that are still relatively not well understood.

There are different states of reduced consciousness. Clouding of consciousness is when someone has a mildly altered mental state, with inattention and reduced wakefulness. A confusional state is a more profoundly altered mental state, with disorientation and difficulty following commands. Lethargy is severe drowsiness, where someone can be roused by moderate stimuli but then will fall back to sleep. Obtundation is worsening lethargy, with drowsiness in between periods of sleep. Stuporose patients need vigorous stimuli to rouse them; left alone, they'll lapse back into unresponsiveness.

The term coma comes from the ancient Greek koma, meaning deep sleep. It denotes unarousable unresponsiveness, where a person is unable to be woken, they fail to respond normally to painful stimuli, they lack a sleep–wake cycle, their brainstem reflexes such as pupil response are depressed, and they do not initiate voluntary actions. The chances of improving from a coma depend very much on its cause. An accidental drug-overdose coma can be reversed if treated promptly. Some people emerge from a coma after years, however, these instances are rare. The depiction of such recoveries in popular media is also often false, showing a person bouncing out of bed, with good muscle bulk, composed and happy. In reality, many survivors may have profound psychological, physical and intellectual difficulties, including speech deficits.

In general, many cases of non-iatrogenic (not caused by medical treatment) coma are due to drug or alcohol intoxication or overdose. Other causes include: cardiac arrest, leading to low oxygen levels to the brain; stroke, leading to sudden cessation of blood flow to parts of the brain; trauma; hypo- or hyperthermia; sepsis; toxins, such as carbon dioxide from a severe asthma attack; prolonged seizures: and altered blood-sugar levels.

Anaesthetic drugs are used to induce medical comas in patients as a neuro-protective measure (a coma can reduce brain swelling) or to ensure that an operation can proceed smoothly without the patient's awareness. However, most anaesthetists do not tell their patients that they are putting them into a 'reversible coma', as this will cause needless panic; rather, they tell them they are 'putting them to sleep' for a defined period of time. Some anaesthetised patients later recount much of what was said around them while they were supposedly unconscious.

A dying person may lose sight and smell and taste and touch. They may lose knowledge of their own self. Yet many believe that the sense of hearing is the last to go. Jenny says she remembers a young patient who had a large tumour compressing his trachea (windpipe). Even though he was sedated and paralysed, she had an intuition that he was aware of what was happening. There were no objective signs to back this up – no spikes in heart rate or other physical signs of distress – however, she asked the consultant if she could increase the patient's sedation to keep him more comfortable. She also talked constantly to him, telling him what she was doing and why, sharing snippets of daily life with him. When the paralysis was weaned off and the patient woke up, he clutched Jenny's hand. His eyes opened wide, he gave a thumbs-up sign. After he had been extubated, he said he'd thought he was dead. The only thing that stopped him from giving up was the voice of an 'Aussie girl' that kept reassuring him he was okay, that his kids were okay.

Other patients who have recovered from comas describe watching spectacular ice-and-light shows in Alaska; meanwhile, in the real world, ice packs were being applied to their bodies. Many describe waiting in a white room or entering a white tunnel and not knowing who they were waiting for. Many also say they heard or felt things that were happening in the real world – a nurse washing their hair, relatives holding their hands and weeping. Sometimes these occurrences became weirdly distorted in their minds.

***

Was Mario aware of his family's pleas? Or were his involuntary movements imbued with extra significance by desperate relatives?

In cases of toxic-metabolic brain injury, such as that due to liver or kidney failure, various involuntary abnormal movements can be observed. One such movement is asterixis, where the wrist is extended, resembling a bird flapping its wings. This could perhaps explain the movement Mario's family interpreted as him pointing towards heaven.

Certainly Jenny has never forgotten Mario's death. She knows the 'benediction' helped resolve a clinical impasse. It brought closure for the family. And that in itself is significant.

Jenny continues to provide all her patients with the same outstanding care that impressed the British prime minister so much. But she is now particularly mindful of always talking to her unconscious patients, reassuring them, providing that human connection in the midst of a bewildering and traumatic time. After all, she reasons, you never know who might be listening.

One bullet, one man

patient: Ahmed; rehabilitation specialist: Dr Amy Donald

There are some people who are so inherently hopeful and resilient that they seem to recover from personal tragedy at a phenomenal rate. Even if the initial trauma they experience is shocking and painful. Even if their lives will never be the same again. Ahmed is such a patient. In this account, he has chosen to use his real first name, but not his last name; he is protective of his family.

For Dr Amy Donald*, his rehabilitation specialist, Ahmed's recovery from extensive trauma verges on the spectacular. It confirms for her the powerful ways in which hope can heal and restore. The thirteenth-century poet Rumi wrote: 'The moon stays bright when it doesn't avoid the night'; for Dr Donald, it is the accelerative effect of acceptance, of not 'avoiding the night' that is trauma or pain, which can make the difference to a patient's recovery.

***

On 15 March 2019, Ahmed gathers with other worshippers for Friday prayers at the Linwood mosque in Christchurch. Autumn is in full swing. The streets are carpeted with a layer of fallen leaves – cherry reds, citric yellows. Lunchtime traffic is busy, crawling along roads still scarred by the Christchurch earthquakes a decade prior.

The mosque is a humble wooden building. It started life as a Sunday School hall, and then became a community centre, before being turned into Christchurch's second mosque in 2018. Brown carpet patterned with geometric shapes lines the floor, a brightly lit chandelier lifts the eyes to the heavens. The walls are adorned simply, with framed passages from the Koran. The smell of spicy mutton curry wafts through the building from the small kitchen; lunch will be shared after prayers. The New Zealand Muslims who gather here originate from all over the world: Afghanistan, Malaysia, India, Pakistan, Indonesia. They are shopkeepers, doctors, lawyers, bankers.

Ahmed hails originally from Hyderabad, a bustling city in south-central India. He's a quiet, thoughtful man, with a salt-and-pepper goatee, an introspective demeanour. Common to many other New Zealanders of Indian origin, Ahmed is multilingual. His first language is Urdu, but he also speaks English, Hindi and Telegu. He was brought up in the Muslim faith and tries to abide by its tenets of fasting, prayer and looking after others. He says he remembers how New Zealand felt 'like heaven on earth' when he first arrived in 2008. All the space, the green forests and fields, the air that smelt of oxygen and bright sunshine. After pumping petrol at a gas station and other jobs, Ahmed found a position managing a Christchurch restaurant. He experienced some racism here in New Zealand, yet he doesn't think it affected him too much. It was all 'relatively mild'. This belies the experiences of other Muslims in New Zealand, particularly female Muslims, who are often more visibly different.

On this particular Friday, as Ahmed and his friends kneel for prayers in the Linwood mosque, they hear an odd sound. A *rat-a-tat*, a ricochet of metal and broken glass. The sound may be common in movies, but no one in the mosque recognises it at first as gunfire. It is so out of place in the quiet suburbia of Christchurch that they continue praying. It is 1.52 pm.

An imam looks out of the first-floor window. He does a double take then starts shouting, 'Quick, everyone, someone is shooting outside!'

Still the worshippers do not move – the words make no sense in this country. This is not America – where there's been more than 110 mass shootings since 1982; where a toddler can accidentally kill their mother with a loaded gun left lying in her handbag – this is New Zealand, named the second most peaceful country in the world by the Global Peace Index in 2019. So it is not until gunshots hit the windows that panic ensues.

Ahmed is kneeling in the last row of male worshippers. He turns to the women behind him and instructs them to head downstairs and stay there. The shooting stops for a moment, and Ahmed steps out into the main hall to assess the situation. The shooter, dressed in black, is standing just outside the door. Police will later recover six guns from him, with illegal modifications. So much weaponry to bolster himself against unarmed men, women and children. The man sees Ahmed, points his gun and fires his last bullet, then drops the empty gun. Ahmed feels the fierce punch of a bullet hitting his right collarbone. The shockwave from the bullet ripples through his flesh, stuns him.

As the shooter retreats to get another gun, Afghani worshipper Abdul Aziz chases the assailant with a credit-card-reader machine and throws it at him. Aziz then finds one of the discarded guns and throws this at the shooter's windscreen, shattering the glass. He screams at the man as he pursues him. Aziz will later say in interviews and in court that he saw real fear in the shooter's face. The gunman drives off, thwarted from further aggression. The attack has lasted three minutes.

Ahmed has fallen to the ground. Initially, he feels no pain; he is in shock and disbelief. His right shoulder area feels hot and wet, mangled. His mouth fills with blood. His arm is not working normally and hangs from his body like a dead weight. Ahmed's wife is hysterical. She tries to drag him backwards into the female section of the mosque. She is cut by pieces of glass, trampled by others.

'I thought I was going to die,' says Ahmed. 'I was losing so much blood that I was struggling to stay awake. I asked my wife to look after our kids. I told her that I didn't think I was going to survive this.'

After about five minutes, police enter the mosque. Some of them are in plain clothes, which frightens the survivors further until they realise these people are police officers. Paramedics are next on the scene and they rapidly triage the injuries. There is a river of blood on the floors of the mosque. So much so that all the carpet will need to be ripped up later and refurbished. Due to the severity of his injury, Ahmed is deemed high priority and is transported to Christchurch Hospital in the second ambulance that arrives. He struggles to maintain consciousness. When he finally reaches the hospital, he passes out and wakes up four days later.

As the chain of events becomes clearer, it emerges that the gunman first entered nearby Al-Noor mosque and shot people, before driving to Linwood mosque. Fifty-one people (47 men and 4 women) die from the attacks, a further 49 are injured. Many of the victims are the primary breadwinners for their families, and all leave behind traumatised, frightened relatives.

***

Friday starts like any other day in Christchurch Hospital's emergency department – kids who've fallen off jungle gyms, a patient writhing with a kidney stone, a man rushed in with chest pain. The scene changes dramatically as multiple ambulances turn up with gunshot victims. Relatives and friends bring others who are stable enough to travel by car. A four-year-old girl needs CPR; she will remain in a coma for weeks. Within 45 minutes, the department fills up with 50 patients. One person dies in ED. It begins to look like a war zone: a maelstrom of resus trolleys, gurneys, plastic tubing, crying patients and their relatives. Orthopaedic, plastics and cardiothoracic surgeons are called to assist. Patients are sent to the radiology department for scans, and then sent straight to the operating theatre – there's not enough space in ED for them to come back. The postoperative recovery area is opened up to accommodate patients.

Ahmed has a gunshot wound to his right upper chest. Imaging reveals a scatter zone of bullet fragments through his flesh; he will need multiple operations over many months to remove residual fragments. The wound is still actively bleeding, and his oxygen saturations are dropping. In ED, two chest drains are inserted to remove blood.

He's then rushed to theatre. An emergency clamshell thoracotomy prises open his ribcage so that the surgeons can assess his injuries. He's got a right collarbone fracture; it is comminuted (in multiple pieces) and compound (there's a break in the skin near the fracture). A cement spacer is inserted into the fracture site as a temporary measure. This is made of bone cement and impregnated with antibiotics; it will help the soft tissues around the injury keep their shape until definitive surgery later on. In the next few days, weeks and months, Ahmed will have many revisions of this fractured clavicle and trimming of the cement spacer to fit. Eventually he will have a bone graft for his damaged collarbone taken from his iliac crest (the curvy pelvic bone that juts out on either side of the lower abdomen).

There's a large haematoma around the fracture, but neither the nearby subclavian artery nor vein are bleeding at this point. Ahmed also has a bruise to the upper lobe of his right lung. He has a significant injury to his brachial plexus. This is a collection of nerves arising from the neck that is located in the armpit area. The nerves of the plexus bifurcate and cleave in a complex tapestry to provide power and sensation to the arm. The surgeons wonder if he potentially has an injury to his right phrenic nerve as well. One of the most important nerves in the body, this provides the primary motor supply to our diaphragm, and thus helps us to breathe. The surgeons painstakingly clean up the mangled and non-viable tissue, cut out fragments of bullets, repair what they can.

Over the next few months, Ahmed will have multiple operations on these damaged nerves, culminating in sural nerve grafts from the backs of both legs as attempted replacements. The sural nerve is a common donor in peripheral nerve surgery. It's easily located on the posterolateral aspect of the lower leg, it's easily dissected out, and it is of a good length. However, to date, Ahmed's graft has not fully restored normal function in his right arm.

After his initial surgery, Ahmed is transferred to ICU. He's still hypoxic (low in oxygen levels), so he remains intubated. A CT scan shows that he has likely aspirated debris into his lungs. A bronchoscopy is performed, which shows large volumes of blood in both of his main bronchi, and this is suctioned out as much as possible. He is covered with antibiotics after the fluid suctioned from his trachea grows E. coli. He is also started on clexane, a medication that is injected under the skin and prevents blood clots in immobile people. However, clexane is not halal, so once Ahmed is alert enough to discuss this, he opts for rivaroxaban tablets instead.

Extensive physiotherapy and occupational therapy help keep his injured arm as limber as possible. Nonetheless, he has little to no movement below shoulder level, and his sensation is only 30 per cent normal.

He is regularly reviewed by the psychiatric liaison team for acute distress and anxiety and ongoing post-traumatic stress disorder (PTSD). Ahmed describes nightmares, flashbacks, trauma-related thoughts and feelings, and difficulty sleeping. The psychological trauma is immense, not just because of his own injuries, but because of the deaths and injuries of so many friends.

Altogether, Ahmed spends two months in hospital, with short visits home to assess his ability to function there. He is then discharged to Burwood Hospital, which has a rehabilitative focus. His mood improves, albeit slowly, and he becomes focused on improving his function. He prefers to keep busy during the day to avoid ruminating on the horrific attack. Staff note that he is at times hypervigilant, and he also displays avoidance behaviour, such as not going out at night.

Relatives fly over from India to help and Victim Support provides financial and other help. He also receives ongoing psychological support, and he makes goals: to be able to return to his role as chairman of the mosque; to return to normal family life; to drive; to manage pain; to heal emotionally.

***

Dr Amy Donald studied medicine at Otago University. As a junior doctor, Amy was assigned to do a stint at the Burwood Spinal Unit. Initially, she dreaded the thought of working there. She was unsure about this sphere of medicine or how she'd cope working with severely injured people, but she ended up loving it. Going on a patient's journey with them, helping them to be the best they could be, finding a pathway forward, providing a modicum of hope: it really suited her. Amy felt like she'd found her place in medicine. She went back as a registrar and trained in Rehabilitation Medicine.

Before Ahmed, there was another patient during her early years as a registrar who showed a similar level of tenacity and hope. 'He was a young man who'd had a cervical spinal-cord injury. He was told early on by one of the acute hospital doctors that he'd be a tetraplegic for life. I met him again two years later. My jaw almost hit the floor when he came into my room. He was on crutches, and although it was a struggle, he was walking. That guy, and Ahmed, reinforce one of the most powerful weapons someone can have at their disposal – hope.

A couple of statements I wish doctors would never say to their patients include "you'll never walk again" or "you'll never get better". Destroying someone's hope is tantamount to destroying any possibility of recovery.'

Amy's provenance nowadays is the long-term care and management of patients with chronic pain, brain and spinal-cord injuries, amputations and orthopaedic trauma. The aim of Rehabilitation Medicine is to maximise independence and to improve quality of life for someone who has had a significant illness or injury. She works with a team of doctors, nurses, physiotherapists, occupational therapists, dietitians and social workers.

***

Amy first meets Ahmed in June 2019, just three months after the shootings. It is helpful for a patient to be referred as early as he is; it increases the input Amy and the team can have into their care. All of Ahmed's consults are covered by ACC, the government organisation that provides compulsory insurance cover for personal injury for everyone in New Zealand, whether they are citizens like Ahmed, residents or even just visitors. ACC is a no-fault scheme that's the only one of its kind in the world. This means that it will cover personal injury even if the person themselves caused the injury. However, it also means that New Zealanders generally can't sue for the costs of the injury or its negative effects.

Right from the start, Amy is struck by how calm Ahmed is in the face of adversity. She notes his remarkable attitude, his drive to get better. 'Even though it was just three months after a significant trauma, Ahmed was quite far down that track of coping. Some people have the ability to get there quickly,' she says. 'Other people take years. Some put on a brave face, but over the course of multiple consults, it becomes obvious if they are pretending – their defences start to crumble. The most vital component of Ahmed's recovery, I think, has been his acceptance. That, and he's adaptable.'

It's well known that acceptance of difficult circumstances is fundamental in allowing someone to move forward. Amy knows only a little about Ahmed's Muslim faith, but she notes how faith can certainly bring purpose, structure, hope and resilience into people's lives, even in the face of inexplicable events. Familial and community support are also vital.

Rehabilitation specialists see people at their best and worst, and in different stages of grief and coping. Amy's modus operandi is firstly to sit with a patient and to listen, to learn about them as a person. This consultation can take up to two hours. Follow-up consults are about 30–45 minutes long. Amy allows the patient to explain how they are feeling, how they are coping. She finds out about their pre-injury levels of function and the important things they enjoy doing. Then, together with the patient, she helps develop realistic goals.

Ahmed has already had extensive and repeat surgery by the time he arrives in Amy's office. He still has shrapnel peppered through his flesh. The surgeons have, in the end, decided to leave these as they are wedged in too deep. He is on a stable cocktail of pain medication: pregabalin, tramadol, nortriptyline, methadone and the humble paracetamol. Amy works with Ahmed to optimise these medications and reduce them where possible.

His brachial-plexus injury is so extensive that, to this day, Ahmed's right arm can barely move. Because of the motor dysfunction and weakness, it drags and feels heavy. He wears a sling to help carry the weight of it. His left arm gets sore also, due to overuse. As well as ongoing weakness, Ahmed has persistent neuropathic pain. This occurs with chronic degenerative nerve disease (in poorly controlled diabetes or multiple sclerosis, for example). It can also occur due to alcoholism, vitamin B deficiency, viral illnesses such as shingles, vascular malformations, chemotherapy or cancer. Phantom limb pain is an uncommon cause of neuropathic pain: the brain thinks it's receiving pain signals from an amputated body part (in reality, the nerves proximal to the amputation are misfiring). In some patients, no actual cause for neuropathic pain is found.

Typically, non-neuropathic pain (or nociceptive pain) is due to a specific injury or illness. If you stub your toe or drop a brick on your foot, your nerves immediately send complaining tweets to your brain. With neuropathic pain, the nerves are so damaged on an ongoing basis, they fire off pain signals to the brain with no prompting. Hence, such a patient may be sitting doing nothing and suddenly get bouts of severe pain.

This might be chronic and unrelenting or intermittent. It is often described as intense, shooting, burning pain, sometimes with associated numbness of the affected part, sometimes with hypersensitive skin. There may be a loss of ability to detect temperature. It can become hard to wear constrictive clothing – even the slightest pressure could cause the neuropathic pain to start, like a discordant clanging symphony in skin and muscle. Simple non-painful activities such as brushing hair or standing in a cold area can become painful.

Neuropathic pain can also worsen with time. Because an individual's pain is invisible to others, it can be hard to describe exactly what it feels like, or how much it affects daily life. It can be hard to control. Pain is complex, and different for different people, and it is sometimes overlaid with anxiety, depression and fatigue. 'Brachial plexus neuropathic pain is often said to be the worst pain one can experience,' Amy says. 'Ahmed describes his right palm as feeling like it's in a burning fire. Ahmed also experiences similar pain in the triceps area.'

Typically, non-steroidal anti-inflammatory drugs such as ibuprofen don't help neuropathic pain. Opiates such as codeine and morphine are not as effective as they could be. Anti-epileptics such as gabapentin and carbamazepine, or tricyclic antidepressants such as amitriptyline can help; sometimes nerve blocks such as injected anaesthetic agents may also temporarily help.

Physiotherapists and occupational therapists work with Ahmed. His deltoid muscle function, the muscles on the rounded contour of the shoulder, improves, which helps prevent his shoulder joint from subluxing inferiorly (slipping downwards out of its socket). This helps him to better position his arm in front of him, and reduces muscular discomfort.

'He has some flexion movement of his fingers and wrist,' says Amy. 'If this improves he may develop enough strength to be a candidate for tendon transfer surgery. That could provide him with some hand function.' Physical therapy has also concentrated on management of his good left arm, to stretch and strengthen it so it doesn't become overworked.

Amy is beginning to space out the appointments she has with Ahmed. 'It really is remarkable how well and how quickly he's improved overall. Nonetheless, he still has a long road ahead, with the likelihood that there will be ups and downs and challenges still to come.'

***

For Amy Donald, Ahmed is unforgettable because he accepted the trajectory of that bullet in his body quicker than others may have done, and transformed it by sheer dint of hope and resilience.

Hope, optimism and resilience help people bounce back and even thrive in the face of adversity. Multiple studies have found better health outcomes in patients who either naturally possess, or who receive psychological training to develop, these traits.[1] Hope is described as an optimistic frame of mind that expects positive outcomes, even in the face of contrary evidence. People with high levels of hope are found to have better life satisfaction, with better health, academic and economic outcomes. Some researchers have found that hope can be augmented by strengthening interpersonal relationships, exploring one's faith and learning to control one's symptoms.

Resilience is our ability to bounce back from negative events without succumbing to despair. Resilient individuals typically have an optimistic outlook, high levels of curiosity, positive emotional states and an openness to new experiences. They tend to have good social support, coping strategies, empowerment, hardiness, spirituality, healthy ways of appraising events, an internal locus of control and the ability to positively accept adverse events. They are more likely to engage in health-enhancing behaviours such as exercise and following treatment regimens. They have a coherent world view, and are more 'bendy' – they adapt to change better.

It is important to distinguish between negative acceptance and positive acceptance. The former might be called stoic, or realistic, acceptance, where a patient accepts their diagnosis but then does little else. Think of Eeyore, the morose but sweet donkey from A. A. Milne's Winnie-the-Pooh books. He's a shining example of the sort of stoicism that expects the worst. Some Eeyorisms: 'One can't complain. I have my friends. Someone spoke to me only yesterday.' 'The nicest thing about the rain is that it always stops. Eventually.' Negative acceptance can lead to worse outcomes; for example, decreased survival times and higher rates of treatment of side effects in women with breast cancer.[2] In contrast, positive acceptance sees patients accept their diagnosis and then actively seek to live with it, improve it and, in some circumstances, overcome it. Obviously, not all patients have inherent levels of hope, resilience and active acceptance. For those who don't, psychological training and other support systems can go a long way towards improving outcomes and quality of life.

Until the day of the Christchurch mosque attacks, Ahmed was a hard-working man, a conscientious citizen and a small-business owner. Spending time with his wife and young family was and still is a priority. He used to love going for long drives and walks in the countryside. He has a personality that is intuitively adaptable, a faith that gives him a salient construct of life and a sense of purpose, and a vigorous motivation in his familial obligations.

Life will never be the same again, and there are days when things are a huge struggle. Nonetheless, he has certainly inspired Dr Amy Donald in the remarkable ways he has adapted to his new normal.

Hongi the wairua

patient: Kiri*; kaumātua: Piripi Daniels; psychiatrist:
Dr Andrew Howie

The practice of medicine is both an art and a science. It's possible to learn the science of medicine – over six years of medical school, then for years and years afterwards – with the help of textbooks, clinical practice and the oversight of experienced peers. The art of medicine is more amorphous. It exists in that liminal space between health practitioner and patient, a space that is a lodestone of desire and belief, fraught with potential conflict. It differs from patient to patient, practitioner to practitioner, and even over time between the same practitioner and patient.

A good grasp of the art of medicine is particularly key when a patient's explanation of their symptoms doesn't tally with medical norms. Psychiatrist Dr Andrew Howie is reminded, when he meets patient Kiri*, that the best course of action sometimes is to be cognisant of the limitations of one's own knowledge, bias and experience, and to know when to allow a colleague to take over.

***

Kiri and her partner are driving through a small North Island town on their way to catch up with whānau. It's a spring day in September, the first week of the school holidays. The mighty Waikato River, overhung with cool numinous fog, curves to meet the road, then swings out and further away. Reeds and rushes line the bank, skeletal trees are just starting to burst with life, harakeke trail in the water.

Suddenly there's a flash of colour to their left. A blur of yellow darts out from between the parked cars. Runs out onto the road. *Thud.*

It's the most sickening sound Kiri has ever heard. That unmistakeable sound of metal and soft flesh colliding. Her stomach twists. 'Shit! Was that a kid?'

Kiri's partner screeches to a stop. They both jump out of the car, and race to the front. Kiri is half praying, half trying not to scream. They see a small child spreadeagled on the damp tarmac. He's not moving. His yellow T-shirt has ridden up, exposing his tummy. His right leg, bent at a funny angle, pokes out of his denim shorts; the thigh bone looks odd, swollen.

Kiri kneels beside the boy. She's not sure if he is alive or dead. She learnt some basic first-responder training ages ago but she's never had to use it in real life. Right now, she can't remember a thing. Her brain is frozen with panic.

'Oh shit, oh shit. No, no, no!'

Kiri's partner falls to his knees beside the child. 'Is he alive? Is he breathing? I'll call 111!' He punches the emergency number on his phone. 'C'mon, little buddy, just open your eyes, c'mon!'

Someone on the pavement starts to scream. The screams bring other people running out of a nearby house. They start yelling when they see the boy. Several adults surround Kiri and her partner. An angry clot of words and hot breath. A young woman pushes Kiri away, cradles the boy's head. The woman is sobbing in terror.

'What the hell happened?' yells an older man. He's livid. His eyes pop. He's practically spitting as he speaks.

'The kid just ran out, it was so quick, I couldn't even …'

'You been drinking, buddy?'

'No!'

'You were driving too fast, eh! Weren't you? Eh?'

'Look, man, it was an accident, I swear!'

'If anything happens to my moko, I'm gonna fucken kill you, bro.'

More family members surround them. Someone jabs Kiri's partner's chest, causing him to stumble backwards. He looks at Kiri, frightened. His eyes flick towards their car. Where are the police? The ambulance? The situation is so heated, so volatile, Kiri is not sure what's going to happen next. She backs away from the group, sits in the passenger seat, locks the door.

Another car drives up and pulls over – more relatives have arrived. Kiri's partner uses the distraction to slip back inside the car himself. He throws the car into reverse. The tyres squeal and the couple speed away. They are too scared to hang around. They head straight to Kiri's whānau in Auckland. She's so upset she can't speak at first, then she finally tells her family what happened. They urge Kiri and her partner to go to the police. The car is taken in for forensic examination, to check for damage and for DNA evidence from the victim. The couple are interviewed under caution. Kiri's partner is breath-tested for alcohol. A serious crash unit investigator is dispatched to the scene to examine it and to interview any possible witnesses.

Over the next few weeks, Kiri hides at home. She's a professional Māori woman in her thirties; nothing like this has ever happened to her before. She has nightmares, flashbacks. She hears the sickening thud of the child being crunched by metal. It makes her sit up in bed in the middle of the night. Her heart ricochets inside her ribs, her mouth is dry, her palms sweaty. She replays the scene over and over. The flash of yellow. The fog twisting like pale fingers over the road. The suddenness of it all. Could they have done anything differently? Were they driving too fast?

The child's family now know who Kiri and her partner are. New Zealanders often have just two degrees of separation, but in this part of the country, dotted with small communities, the connections are even more tight-knit. The couple start receiving messages on social media. They learn that the little boy has died in hospital of his injuries. The messages become increasingly unpleasant, threatening. They insinuate harm to Kiri and her family.

Kiri cloisters herself in her room. She barely comes out, even to eat meals. She is unable to attend work. She withdraws from her family. Her mood is persistently low, a suffocating fug of darkness that slithers into her mind and clouds her vision. She cries all day, finds it hard to sleep as it brings awful flashbacks.

Some things that Kiri has never experienced before start to happen. She smells blood, petrol, sticky tarmac, briny water. She feels something cold and prickly 'walking' along her arms. She hears voices muttering around her. Sometimes the voices are not clear in what they are saying, like a radio tuned to low static. But to Kiri, they sound negative, and she is sure they are talking about her. At other times, the voices are clearer, and they are scathing. She sees bizarre figures, large and small, humanoid in appearance, scuttling around the edges of her room. Some of the figures she recognises as her own dead relatives; when the figures approach her, she hides under the bedcovers until they go away.

Her worried family refer her to mental-health services. Her case is taken up by Whītiki Maurea, the Māori Mental Health and Drug & Alcohol Service in north-west Auckland. Whītiki Maurea weaves together Māori healing practices and Western clinical practice. Neither takes precedence. Therapy focuses on the patient's wider whānau, and seeks the best possible health outcomes for Māori using a marae- and wairua- (spirit-) based approach.

Kiri undergoes a cultural assessment, beginning with karakia, waiata, an acknowledgement of her whakapapa and a thorough mental-health assessment. In recognition of the partnership approach of this mental-health service, Kiri is assessed by two practitioners: Dr Andrew Howie, a very experienced Pākehā psychiatrist, and Piripi Daniels, a kaumātua with a wealth of traditional knowledge and societal connections. Piripi Daniels died in 2020. He was a great kauri of a man, who Andrew says taught him much about the fundamental importance of Māori approaches to spiritual and mental health, especially when dealing with Māori patients.

This story of patient Kiri and her distressing descent into mental illness is as much a testament to Piripi's enduring legacy and knowledge as it is about Andrew's recognition that there are 'more things in heaven and earth' than are contained in the *Diagnostic and Statistical Manual of Mental Disorders 5* (DSM-5).

Andrew and Piripi sit with Kiri in an interview room. Kiri is dishevelled, distressed and disorganised. There are dark circles under her eyes. She's lost weight in the four weeks since the accident. Her clothes hang loosely. She probably hasn't showered or changed for a few days. There's a rankness to her, the almost fetid smell of old sweat and fear. Her family have told the team this behaviour is completely out of character. She's normally neatly kept and punctual with her work and family commitments. They're adamant she's not taking drugs as they monitor when she gets up, when she eats, when she sleeps.

Andrew asks Kiri to recount what happened. She does so
haltingly. She stops at times, mid-sentence, lost in thought. She
speaks of the panic attacks she's been having, sometimes in the
middle of the night. She speaks of the nightmares, the visitations
by shadowy threatening figures, the voices that say horrible
things about her. Her mood is labile. Her eyes bloom with fresh
tears, then just as quickly she switches to anger, then fear. She
glances sideways, looks over Andrew's shoulder and cocks her
head, frowning. She's listening to something that Andrew can't
hear or see.

'It was clear to me,' Andrew says, 'that Kiri was displaying
symptoms of psychosis, and responding to auditory and visual
hallucinations. I had started to formulate possible diagnoses
as she spoke: perhaps post-traumatic stress disorder with
dissociation, perhaps a brief psychotic episode with stressors,
perhaps a panic disorder or a major depressive disorder. But
about halfway through the interview, I noticed that Piripi had
started to behave oddly as well. That threw me a bit. I'd never
seen him like this before. I thought, gosh, what's he doing?'

The usually calm kaumātua is darting his eyes this way and
that. He, too, looks over Andrew's and Kiri's shoulders as they
speak and looks surprised, perplexed. Andrew stops to ask Piripi
what is happening. 'I can see small creatures out of the periphery
of my vision, Andrew,' Piripi says. 'I think this is a mate Māori
issue. Do you mind if I take over in te reo?'

Mate Māori is the term for an illness that is thought to be
psychosomatic, and often precipitated by transgressions of tapu

or mākutu. Tapu has various meanings: sacred, prohibited, restricted, set apart, forbidden. Mākutu refers to sorcery or witchcraft. More on this later.

Andrew's vocabulary of te reo Māori extends to about 100 words, so he cannot fully follow the ensuing conversation between Piripi and Kiri. However, Kiri seems a lot more engaged than she did when speaking with Andrew. She is listening intently to Piripi. He even coaxes a small, timorous smile out of her.

Piripi says to Andrew, 'My initial suspicions are right, I think. This is not a hinengaro [mind] or tinana [body] issue. It's partly a whānau issue. It's most definitely about wairua. I'd like to arrange a meeting between Kiri and her whānau and elders from her tribe. After that, we should try to meet with the child's family and the elders from their tribe also.' Piripi closes the interview with a heartfelt karakia. He then takes over Kiri's care, and Andrew hears that the proposed meetings have been organised.

A month later, Andrew has a consultation with a young, well-dressed woman. Kiri is smiling and personable, poised and articulate. She has good affect, good eye contact. She displays no symptoms of psychosis. She explains how Piripi said she needed to put right what had gone wrong through karakia, a meeting with the child's whānau and a clear apology. Her symptoms resolved after she had addressed her transgression and the pain of the bereaved, once she had recognised her symptoms in the holistic context of Māori spirituality, and given space to make amends.

Kiri's story was Andrew's first encounter with mate Māori. He feels he could so easily have misdiagnosed her using Western phenomenology and given her a psychiatric label and drugs. It was a powerful reminder to him to step back and let someone else lead.

***

Andrew Howie would say respectful partnership runs in his genes. His ancestors arrived in New Zealand in 1823, having sailed here from Australia – possibly one of the first twenty or so European families in New Zealand. His paternal great-grandfather, Reverend Arthur John Seamer, was a Methodist minister among Māori tribes in the central North Island from 1905. He spoke fluent Māori, was known for his tolerant approach to the beliefs of others, and worked with many tribes, including Te Arawa and Tainui. He also worked alongside the prophet Tahupōtiki Wiremu Rātana, who founded the Rātana church. In the 1990s, Andrew also undertook theological training. This was his first exposure to Māori and Pasifika world views, and to different ways of interpreting spiritual or physical ailments. Later, he worked as a psychiatrist at Broken Hill, with the Barkindji Native Australian tribe in the Darling River basin, New South Wales. Whenever a Barkindji person presented with unusual symptoms, Andrew found it was helpful to ask someone more knowledgeable if the symptoms were congruent with the patient's cultural context.

Andrew and Piripi worked together for five years at Whītiki Maurea. Piripi saw the interface between the physical and the spiritual as porous rather than well-caulked. Kiri's case was not the first time Piripi could 'see' the creatures tormenting a patient. He said he didn't seek them out, as such, but thought that perhaps he was spiritually attuned enough to see them. Piripi encouraged Andrew and others to dwell with uncertainty. 'Hongi the wairua, Andrew,' he would tell him. 'Hongi the wairua.'

***

Diagnosis is only sometimes black and white; it is more often shifting shades of grey, varying according to patient or practitioner or disease. Subjectivity and bias can occur. Take a common condition such as migraine, or a less common but crippling condition such as chronic pain. Both lack conclusive diagnostic testing, yet they are real to those who suffer from them. Clinical medicine has correctly identified and described conditions long before diagnostic tests became available, for example, epilepsy, Parkinson's disease or Huntington's disease (the latter described and diagnosed for 110 years before its genetic basis was uncovered).

In the field of psychiatry, the art rather than the science of medicine can dominate. It is difficult to be fully objective about parameters as nebulous as someone else's thoughts, feelings, sensations or motivations. The brain is increasingly well mapped, but the mind continues to be an elusive entity, identifiable only by the shadows it casts, rather than by a physical, fleshly presence.

As expertise grows in areas such as brain imaging, genetics, environmental impact and neurophysiology, it is likely that we will see more evidence for the aetiology (causes) of mental illnesses such as psychosis, mania, obsessive-compulsive disorder and crippling anxiety. For now, there remains an element of subjectivity in psychiatric diagnosis. Depending on the century in which a person claimed to be hearing voices, they could have been labelled a prophet, a heretic or a schizophrenic. Cultural differences and social and psychological factors can all alter the presentation of the same illness in different people. Studies have noted, for example, that indigenous people and ethnic minorities are more at risk of being diagnosed, and sometimes misdiagnosed, as schizophrenic by Western-trained psychiatrists.[3]

For Kiri, both culture and spirituality played a part. The accident and subsequent death of the child, and the family's ensuing anger, served to disrupt her spiritual and cultural equilibrium, leading to distressing emotional and mental sequelae. One possible explanation for her symptoms is a culture-bound syndrome: a type of illness displaying both bodily and psychiatric symptoms, recognised as a disease process only within a specific society or culture. For example, individuals who have 'amok' in Malay culture display violent behaviour and persecutory ideas in response to extreme stress; in Samoan culture, 'ma i fasia' involves hallucinations and unusual behaviour in those who are believed to have grieved spirits; and so on. Essentially, various ethnic populations have different ways of responding to conflict or stressful situations. Behaviour in a person that is seen as unacceptable in Western society may lead to a psychiatric diagnosis by a Western-trained clinician while it may be seen as a normal adaptive response to a stressful situation in the person's own culture, and handled without resorting to medication. Piripi Daniels recognised Kiri's presentation as being congruent with a Māori world view, a fundamentally Māori response to a traumatic incident.

Another aspect to Kiri's presentation is spirituality. Māori culture has always recognised spirituality as an intrinsic part of hinengaro. However, Western psychiatry has tended to ignore or pathologise spiritual experiences and religion. Someone undergoing a 'spiritual emergency' may be disoriented, fearful, have disordered moods and experience hallucinations and delusions in response to a traumatic experience; the content of the psychotic experiences tends to revolve around spiritual themes (encounters with mythological beings, for example, as in Kiri's case).[4] Assessing the patient by recognising his or her particular belief systems and values has been shown to lead to faster and more comprehensive recovery; Christian- and Muslim-based psychotherapy, for example, has led to better recovery from anxiety symptoms in certain patients. The authors of this study note: 'One of the major factors identified as facilitating recovery is hope. Many patients say that spirituality plays a vital role for them in bringing hope, empowerment, identity, and a sense of purpose and meaning.' More research needs to be done to ascertain how spiritual emergencies and culture-bound syndromes overlap with psychosis.

There are connections within te ao Māori to the spiritual and natural worlds, in concepts such as mauri, wairua, tapu, noa and mana. Mauri has been described as an essential life force, the 'bonding element that holds the fabric of the universe together'.[5] Mauri binds someone's wairua, their soul, to their physical being. Should their mauri become noa, or defiled, then a person's physical, intellectual and spiritual welfare is in danger. Noa is often explained as 'common'. Tapu, conversely, is 'sacred' or 'spiritually restricted'. Tapu begins at birth, and refers to the potential of a person; mana is the fulfilment of that potential. Someone with mana has spiritual authority and power.

Traditionally, Māori illnesses were believed to be either mate atua (sickness caused by the gods) or mate tangata (sickness due to physical causes). After European arrival, mate atua became known as mate Māori. The treatment of the latter was particularly via a tohunga (in this context, a healer or priest).

It is quite plausible that some psychiatrists are misdiagnosing Māori with mental-health issues. For example, delusions and hallucinations have been recorded among those experiencing mate Māori. Patterns of speech can be metaphorical in some Māori people, rippling out towards larger ideas. This can be misconstrued as tangential thinking. Even a lack of eye contact can be misinterpreted as a mood disorder, when it actually might indicate whakamā (shame). The concept for the Māori kaupapa centre Whītiki Maurea came about after a psychiatric conference Andrew Howie attended, where Dr Allister Bush, a child and adolescent psychiatrist, and Wiremu NiaNia, a Māori healer and tohunga, both spoke. The pair were developing a framework of Western-based psychiatric practice alongside traditional Māori concepts of mental well-being. They argued that this duality of practice allowed good cultural and clinical assessment and helped build rapport with Māori whānau.

Psychiatrist and professor of Māori studies Dr Mason Durie was also present. For more than four decades, Dr Durie has spearheaded a transformational approach to Māori health. Dr Durie rose and addressed the speakers, and Andrew transcribed Dr Durie's words that day. They are words that still inform his practice today:

> So I just want to say the example that you two have set is an example for all sorts of services. From two pathways you haven't tried to merge them into one pathway. It reminded me of when I was a house surgeon, the year after I graduated, there was a girl who lived at the hospital with viral encephalitis, a Māori girl, and her grandfather came and used to look after her. I knew the grandfather, and we were talking one day and he said he thought he knew of the cause of the viral encephalitis, and I asked him, 'Well, what do you think caused it?' and he said, 'My grand-daughter is affected with mākutu. There is trouble in the family, and this is the result.'

And then he asked me, 'What do you think caused it?' I said with great confidence, 'It was a virus.' And he said, 'Did you see it?' and I said, 'Well, no, I didn't.'

'Did you touch it? Taste it? Smell it?'

'No,' I admitted, and he said, 'Doctor, I admire your faith in the power of unseen things and mysterious forces'. I was translating his mākutu into medical terms, and he was translating my medical terms into spiritual terms. And the worst thing psychiatrists can do, with spiritual experience, is to skip through the DSM until they find a diagnosis. It's a different system. We ought not to explain one system with the tools of the other. They are parallel systems and that is what has been important about this story. You have kept the parallel streams going, not trying to explain one by the other, and I think that is a really good example for all of us.

In accepting that Kiri displayed a complex interplay of symptoms and beliefs that were fully understood within a Māori mental-health framework, not a Western one, Andrew reflects: 'The lingering impression for me is of a world I didn't understand, and the contribution that someone who *did* understand that world could make. Piripi made the correct diagnosis and he brought about a resolution for Kiri that was swift and thorough, and which did not include the use of a diagnostic label or drugs.'

PART 2

The things we carry

A born survivor

patient: Harlow; mother: Justine Brooker;
neonatal nurse: Carole Dunn

It doesn't matter how little you are. If you possess a spark of gutsy determination, if you're in the right place at the right time and surrounded by the right people, you can still make a difference.

In Wellington, there lives a young boy who, had he been born in a different era, would not be alive today. He will always carry the legacy of his traumatic birth, yet his story is one of overcoming insurmountable odds, of thriving and, without being aware of it, of markedly affecting those looking after him.

When Justine Brooker thinks about her last-born son, Harlow, who slipped into the world after just 24 weeks of pregnancy, she remembers a roller-coaster of emotions. Feelings of helplessness, vulnerability, fear. Of depending upon others so much that it hurt to breath. Of feeling so distant from this tiny speck of humanity inside his incubator. A mere fledgling of a child, who sprouted wires like raggedy feathers and who needed so much more assistance and care than most other infants. Justine remembers all those long months of waiting and hoping and praying that Harlow would grow, would improve, would go home.

The old saying that it takes a village to raise a child is even more true for premature babies. Harlow's parents, Justine and Richard, already have three older boys, and so an additional child would have taken skilful juggling, regardless. However, the vagaries of extreme prematurity made everything so much harder with Harlow. Richard wrote on his blog: 'I don't know really how to describe it. In terms even I can understand, we have been through hell. The life of a prem baby is a hard one. On everyone. There is so much pain, fear and misery that at times it nearly overwhelms you. What used to be simple and easy is now like trying to balance an anvil on the tip of a needle.'

The stories of premature infants are inextricably linked to the neonatal staff who care for them. In baby Harlow's case, neonatal nurse Carole Dunn was a vital member of his village, not only looking after him while he was in hospital but also rescuing his parents from drowning in a sea of sleeplessness, feeding difficulties and frustration once Harlow went home.

But Harlow gives as good as he gets. This wee chap has been instrumental in changing his mother's vocation – Justine is now a part-time operations manager for the Neonatal Trust – and instrumental in changing the way post-hospital care is delivered to ex-neonatal-unit babies and their families. Even after all these years (Harlow is now 11), nurse Carole remembers Harlow well. She sees a clear demarcation in her approach: the Before Harlow and After Harlow methods of providing care.

Harlow is clearly quite the mover and shaker, for someone so little.

***

Justine's fourth pregnancy is a total surprise; with three rambunctious boys under the age of seven (each of whom were born a little early, at 36, 35 and 34 weeks respectively), she and her husband are already very busy. However, they are delighted with the news that they will become parents once more. But when Justine has a significant bleed at six weeks, and her serum HCG (pregnancy hormone) levels fall, she assumes she's had a miscarriage. In the weeks that follow, she still doesn't feel 'back to normal' and she heads off to see her GP for another blood test.

'Well, this is a surprise,' her GP says. 'You're still pregnant, Justine!'

Her HCG levels start to rise again. A scan at eight weeks confirms a viable pregnancy with the discovery of a tiny heartbeat, as well as a probable twin that has died in utero, as evidenced by an empty foetal sac floating nearby.

Justine continues to bleed on and off. Each time she wonders if this is it, if this is the end of this precarious pregnancy. She is recommended bed rest from 13 weeks onwards. Bed rest! A monumental undertaking and a ridiculous thing to ask when there are three small children tearing around the house. Yet, rest in bed she does, hoping against hope to save this pregnancy. Justine perseveres till 19 weeks, when the bleeding finally seems to stop. Her obstetric specialist (Justine is under the care of the high-risk antenatal team) suggests that she can cautiously start doing a few things again.

At 21 weeks and two days, Justine has a massive bleed. An ambulance rushes her to Wellington Hospital, and an assessment reveals that her waters have broken. This is not good news. Usually, a baby is well cushioned inside the fluid-filled amniotic sac. The amniotic fluid is made mostly from the mother's plasma, but also partially made up of urine from the foetus. It contains nutrients for the growing foetus, it allows the foetal gut to develop properly, and it provides space and room for limbs and muscles to grow. When the sac breaks prematurely, the baby is at risk of infection, birth injuries and umbilical cord compression, among other dangers.

Justine is admitted to the ward. She is started on intravenous antibiotics to prevent infection affecting herself or the baby. At 23 weeks she goes into labour, and this is artificially delayed for one week with a tocolytic (a medicine that slows or halts labour) in order to allow Harlow to reach just one more week of gestation. It's an important threshold for a baby, this 24-week date. Life outside the womb at 24 weeks is still pretty damn hard, but viability is much improved from what it would be at 23 weeks.

Justine is also given corticosteroids – synthetic versions (dexamethasone or betamethasone) of natural steroids – normally released later on in pregnancy. These help the baby's lungs, gut, and cardiovascular and immune systems to mature, all of which don't fully develop until after 36 weeks of pregnancy. (Steroid treatment was discovered by two New Zealand scientists, Sir Mont Liggins and Ross Howie, in 1972. Initial research was conducted on sheep at Cornwall Park, near National Women's Hospital. Steroid treatment for threatened preterm labour is now international best practice. Babies of mothers who receive this are less likely to die, and less likely to have severe lung disease and other health problems after birth.)

An ultrasound scan at 24 weeks reveals that the amniotic fluid around Harlow has reduced substantially, but that he is still doing okay. Six days later, Justine again goes into labour.

It is 2.30 am on a chilly spring night when Richard receives a call from the midwife. 'Come now. Your wife needs you asap. Baby's on its way!' Thanks to a web of family and friends – invisible in this chapter but an invaluable source of support to Richard and Justine – he is able to leave immediately. Someone else will look after Harlow's three brothers as they sleep.

The entire labour lasts 45 minutes. Justine pushes once and Harlow pops into the world, bottom first, with little fanfare and next to no noise. He doesn't cry. He weighs just 725 grams – as heavy as a bag of grapes – but with skin so devoid of fat it is translucent, scribbled with delicate veins. The neonatal team swoop on Harlow and whisk him away to the neonatal intensive care unit (NICU). Justine's husband arrives 15 minutes too late for the birth of his son.

NICU will be Harlow's home for the next six months. The unit is always warm for little humans, however, it can be uncomfortably warm for big humans. The staff pad around in soft shoes and scrubs. The lights are muted and artificial; no harsh sunlight here, no gusts of fresh oxygen from outdoors. The corridors are lined with lots of high-tech equipment. There's the constant low hum of beeps, whooshes, quiet conversations.

The start of parenthood is always fraught with change. Multiply that umpteen times and you get a sense of the difficulty of having a child in NICU. Everything is recorded, including how much breast milk a mother produces. Everything is noted down. It can feel like you're being graded on your performance. At home, you can pad around in your pyjamas and take naps when you want to, but there's much less privacy in a hospital. Parents have so little control over the safety and health of their infant. Neonatal staff are aware of the stressful, artificial environment that parents face, and they go above and beyond to help.

When Justine and Richard finally get to visit Harlow, he is in an incubator, lying on his back on soft bedding. His skin is pink, like a boiled prawn. There's a tube, secured in place with plasters, that reaches into his trachea and helps him to breathe. There are catheters threaded through his umbilical vessels, bringing him sustenance and important medications. A pulse oximeter is strapped to his right hand; a cool red light shines through his skin, illuminating his flesh with a florid glow. His nappy lies open for now; it looks huge, designed for a larger baby. Justine disinfects her hands and proffers her little finger to Harlow. He clutches it. Harlow is so little that he can be comfortably held in one adult hand.

Harlow's pink colour is a good sign. He moves his arms and legs around, also a good sign. He is soon breathing on his own. However, on day four, the NICU team notes that his abdomen looks swollen and tense, like a dusky melon. X-rays reveal free air inside his abdominal cavity. The medics suspect Harlow has necrotising enterocolitis (NEC), a condition that mainly affects preterm infants, whereby bacteria invade the intestinal wall causing inflammation, infection and damage. Sections of the gut can die, allowing air to escape into the abdominal cavity. Up to 10 per cent of premature infants with very low birth weight (i.e. birth weight less than 1500 grams) may develop this condition.

Two soft rubber drains are inserted through cuts into Harlow's tiny abdominal wall to let the trapped air and mucky intestinal leakage drain out. He is started on antibiotics and intravenous fluids; feeds via his nasogastric tube are temporarily stopped to allow his gut to heal. He is put on a ventilator until his infection markers settle after a week or so, and he is weaned off.

A brain scan picks up a Grade 1 bleed in Harlow's brain. Although this is a low-grade bleed, it may still have consequences for his later development. Fortunately, the bleed does not expand over the next few days.

Four weeks after being admitted to hospital, and six days after Harlow's birth, Justine finally goes home. It's a relief for husband Richard and for the other boys to have her home again. Dad's cooking won't need to be inflicted on anyone anymore. But now starts the juggle of home, work, school and dashing to NICU for Harlow time.

At two weeks old, Harlow's parents cuddle him for the first time. Just one parent at a time, and on different days, and not for very long to avoid tiring him out. There are so many tubes and monitors to navigate, so many alarming beeps, so much paraphernalia. 'I found it hard to bond with Harlow,' says Justine. 'It was just so different to all my other pregnancies.'

The next weeks and months segue into gains and losses. Harlow's weight doubles in seven weeks, thanks to expressed breast milk and top-up feeds. He passes the magical 1-kilo mark, and so his intravenous nutrition feeds can start to decrease. He gets regular transfusions, small thimblefuls of life-giving blood to replace the blood constantly being taken out for various tests. And it is a thimbleful: he receives just 11 millilitres at a time. Sometimes he screams and flails his limbs; at other times he stares beady-eyed at the walls of his incubator. Richard says that he is by turns sweet and delightful, at other times fractious.

Christmas Day sees nurses dressed as angels, lots of toys, and a visit from Harlow's three excited siblings who ogle their little brother through the plastic walls of the incubator. They are enchanted with this small human. They can look but they can't touch at this stage. Back home, they have started to help around the house without being asked, just like little angels themselves. Harlow sails through Christmas and New Year. Just a few days later, however, he crashes. He is as floppy-limbed as a small frog. His heart rate and oxygen levels plummet. Infection is thought to be the culprit. A team of four nurses work on him for hours. They are calm and composed and competent. Harlow is ventilated again.

Two months later, he is off his ventilator. It has been a long hard slog. Everything is recorded in minutiae. Harlow is finally deemed stable enough to be discharged. He has by this stage spent 111 days in NICU. It's the doctors who decide if the baby is well enough to go home; it's the nurses who decide if the parents are ready to manage at home.

Harlow's discharge summary is a litany of the manifestations of extreme prematurity. Chronic lung disease and a pulmonary haemorrhage (bleed in the lung). Suspected necrotising enterocolitis. A patent ductus arteriosus (the hole between the two upper chambers of the heart that allows foetal blood flow to bypass the lungs in utero, but which normally closes after birth. Harlow is given several shots of a medicine designed to close this hole, but it stubbornly refuses to close). Anaemia. Jaundice. Retinopathy of prematurity (abnormal growth of blood vessels in the eye, which can cause visual problems or even blindness).

Harlow only lasts one day at home, and returns to NICU the next day. He is not feeding well, keeps dozing off instead. It is disappointing for the family, but completely in keeping with the 'one step forward, two steps back' journey he has led them on so far. Over the next month, he goes back and forth between home and NICU. He is at times on low-flow oxygen, at other times on different types of ventilation. Harlow is exhausted by the simple act of feeding, and he squawks and complains when something is placed in his mouth. Richard and Justine become increasingly tired and sleep-deprived. Because Harlow tires so easily, and because he is hooked up to so much stuff, the family can't go on any outings. They reach a low point.

When Carole and the team take Harlow back to NICU on 23 April, it is ostensibly for a few days. However, they are alarmed at how burnt out the family is and believe Harlow's parents need respite care. Hence, Harlow is managed in NICU for three weeks instead. This nadir in family life is the catalyst for change. After Harlow, there will be a nationwide shift in how post-hospital care is arranged for neonatal-unit babies. Meanwhile, Harlow's parents sleep and replenish their energy. They all go out for an ice cream for the first time in months. Glimmers of normality hover on the horizon.

***

Nurse Carole Dunn was born in Palmerston North. Her father was a manager in an oil company, so the family moved around a lot – followed the black gold to Alice Springs, Sydney, New Zealand. In sixth form, Carole had a stint of work experience in the Napier intensive care unit for one week. She loved it, and trained as a nurse at Massey University. Carole's aunty remains an influential role model: she is also a nurse and is still working at the age of 75.

After doing some mental-health nursing, Carole worked for eight years for what's known as the 'flight team', helping to retrieve sick neonates from the Wellington Hospital catchment area. She then transitioned into her current role as the neonatal specialty clinical nurse discharge facilitator and has been doing this for almost two decades. This role is more family focused and involves a lot of advocacy. Carole gets great feedback from those she helps.

Wellington NICU has 36 beds and looks after not just premature babies but also any sick term infants (for example, those who are septic, have low blood sugars or who've had a traumatic birth) and surgical infants. The babies and their families originate from anywhere in the central region: Palmerston North, Wanganui, the lower North Island and the top of the South Island, including Nelson and Blenheim.

Before Harlow was born in 2010, there were relatively few extremely premature babies who survived and made it home. Although the neonatal team provided a fantastic in-house service, parents were simply ill-equipped to manage once they were on their own. Almost everything was done for the babies by the medical staff while they were in-patients. It was only near the time of discharge that plans were put in place to transition care to the family. Now, infants are case managed with individualised care plans from day one to provide family-centred care.

'Harlow was unusual in that he was an extremely prem baby who survived, and who also went home with multiple tubes and tanks of oxygen,' says Carole. 'At the time our staff worked hard to look after the medical aspects of a neonate's care, but we didn't have a good handle on each family's psychosocial needs. Harlow's mum, Justine, is such a capable person and she was sure she would be fine, that the minimum skills she'd learnt during her time in neonates would see her through. We all thought she would cope.'

After Harlow had tried to go home several times, but kept being readmitted because of various issues, things came to a head during one of Carole's home visits to check on Harlow's feeding and weight. She says she's so grateful that Justine sat her down that day and was straight up with her. 'She simply said, "Carole, we are not coping. We have three older boys to look after. Our sleep is shot to pieces because Harlow is such a poor feeder. We can't go anywhere as a family and anyway he gets exhausted by even a short trip. We are literally at the end of our tether. Something needs to change."'

Instead of just a home visit, Carole decided to readmit Harlow to give his family a break. This readmission stretched to a three-week respite. Carole started to think holistically in terms of services that could wrap around the family. 'Back then, nothing was available. No care packages, no home help. The plight of high-needs kids and their families was invisible. We were so focused on the tasks that we had to do in hospital, we were too busy to think about how they'd manage afterwards.'

Harlow's GP was a fantastic advocate. Together with Carole, he pushed and pushed for extra support for Justine and her family. Letters were written to the Ministry of Health, and when they were turned down, Carole and the GP persisted. Finally, a package of care was granted that allowed a carer to come in several times a week to help with Harlow's feeds and other support.

This carer made a world of difference to Justine and the family. The pressure-cooker valve was released. Justine could now take her older children to school and kindergarten. She could also connect with her youngest son and spend quality time with him. The family could go on social outings more freely. Harlow ended up having a carer for almost one year, and the carer became an ersatz aunty to the older boys.

Discharge planning for NICU babies now starts upon admission, with care plans and case management. Families are encouraged to be involved in their baby's daily needs and decision-making while in the unit. As long as the baby is well enough, the parents are also encouraged to attend to practical details. Kangaroo care (skin-to-skin contact), shushers (decibel meters that light up if people are speaking too loudly), and 'quiet time' periods are examples of nurse-driven initiatives, medically proven to be effective. It is now also standard practice for many neonatal-unit babies and their families to be offered support packages when they leave hospital, especially if they have unresolved medical issues. Not just in Wellington, but nationwide. Psychosocial needs are identified before discharge and packages can be tailor-made. The Neonatal Trust, where Justine now works, provides this support to families.

'Before Harlow and his family reached crisis point, I was a very task-focused nurse,' says Carole. 'Now, I feel more like a relationship manager. It's so important to have that good connection with babies and their families. Of course, it's vital to help parents learn all the practical stuff, like putting in nasogastric tubes or managing oxygen, but we let them do it at their pace. We aim now to transition care to the family much earlier, and we don't give them a discharge date anymore. Instead, we let them tell us when they are ready to go home. Knowing Harlow has truly been transformational for me.'

***

Worldwide, up to 10 per cent of babies will be born prematurely – before 37 weeks of gestation. That's 15 million babies. In New Zealand, the figure is about 7.4 per cent of all births, or about 4500 babies. Half of these are born before 34 weeks. Extremely preterm babies, like Harlow, are those born before 28 weeks.

According to the World Health Organization, preterm birth complications are the leading cause of death worldwide in children under five years of age. In recent years, this has been as high as 1 million deaths per year. Three-quarters of these deaths (especially in low-income countries) could be prevented with basic interventions, such as good antenatal care, warmth, breast-feeding support and antibiotics. For obvious reasons, there is a dramatic difference in survival rates for preterm babies depending on where they are born.

Survival rates certainly rise steeply the longer a baby manages to stay inside their mother's womb. So much happens with each week of gestation, so much building up of strength and resilience. A premature birth means being born with body systems that are not ready to function independently, and where one system malfunctioning can cause a domino-like collapse in other systems. Of those born at 24 weeks, survival rates are about 50 per cent. Of those who survive, there are often multiple complications. By 28 weeks, survival rates have risen to approximately 90 per cent.

Mere survival is not the end of the story – there are ramifications in later life as well. Even those born just four to six weeks early can suffer from feeding problems and breathing difficulties. The infant brain is one of the last major organs to develop. It is also one of the most fragile, the most easily damaged. At 35 weeks, it will weigh two-thirds of its weight at full term; there is increasing evidence that our brains continue to develop in different ways until we are well into our thirties and forties. Hence, being born early, into an abnormal environment, can lead to significant adverse effects.

In infancy and childhood, ex-prem babies can suffer from increased rates of cerebral palsy, visual and hearing impairments, and poor health and growth. There can be long-term difficulties such as behavioural and social problems, and an increased risk of attention deficit hyperactivity disorder (ADHD) and cot death (sudden infant death syndrome). These children are more likely to require special education services. In adulthood, there will be a higher risk of chronic diseases such as diabetes, hypertension and heart disease.

Preterm births appear to be on the increase worldwide. This is partly due to an increase in fertility treatment, resulting in multiple pregnancies; twin births, for example, can be preterm almost 50 per cent of the time. Other causes are infections such as sexually transmitted infections or other vaginal infections such as bacterial vaginosis; bleeding from the vagina; and developmental abnormalities in the foetus. In most cases, preterm labour is spontaneous, and sometimes no cause is found.

Women who have had a preterm delivery or labour previously are at higher risk of this happening again, as in Justine's case. Other maternal factors associated with a greater risk of preterm delivery include being younger than 18, or over the age of 35 (the latter are more likely to have medical complications such as diabetes or high blood pressure that can cause preterm delivery). Smoking has been a known risk factor for preterm delivery (and stillbirth and cot death) for more than 50 years, however, the exact way in which smoking causes prematurity is not clear. Alcohol, drugs, poor or no antenatal care, domestic violence, lack of social support and stress can all contribute to premature babies. Being very overweight or very underweight as a mother can also contribute.

Certain ethnicities are at higher risk of preterm labour and birth, such as African Americans and Native Americans. In New Zealand, annual perinatal mortality and morbidity figures show that Māori babies are born preterm 8.1 per cent of the time, compared to the national average of 7.4 per cent. Māori babies are also more likely to have a preterm death than Pākehā babies, and it is thought that this is partly due to inequities in antenatal care.

With advances in technology, viability has improved for babies of earlier gestation. In the 1960s, a baby less than 1 kilo in weight, roughly 27 weeks' gestation, was considered non-viable. In the 1970s, viability was possible if an infant was born between 24 and 28 weeks. Today, this has improved to between 23 and 24 weeks.

***

Harlow himself is now doing remarkably well. He has mild cerebral palsy in his left leg and some impaired vision that requires glasses, but not much else. These days, he is mostly a delight to be around, with a cheerful personality and a keen desire to keep up with his older brothers. The impact of his early arrival, however, lives on in the important work carried out by his mother, Justine, and nurse Carole.

A midnight epiphany on childhood

patient: Bopha*; paediatrician: Dr Jin Russell

When an epiphany takes place, it may be powerful enough to change the course of a career. For paediatrician Dr Jin Russell, her epiphany involves a small Cambodian girl called Bopha*.

There's a fistful of epiphanous events scattered throughout history. In the third century BCE, for example, the Greek scholar Archimedes ran through the streets of Syracuse naked, shouting 'Eureka!' ('I have it!'), after he stepped into a bath and realised that the volume of water displaced was equal to the volume of the body part he was submerging. Thus it became possible to accurately measure the volume of an irregularly shaped object.

An epiphany occurs in a fraction of time. A split-second burst of neurons firing and connecting, leading to the revelation of a sublime truth that hitherto eluded us. But there is important groundwork that is laid before this moment. Moments of contemplation, hours of research, the pulling together of disparate strands of experience and knowledge. Then, at a subconscious level, the answer to a problem is found and leaps out at us. We might credit serendipity, we might say 'the universe/God gave it to me' because the insight seems to come from nowhere. We might claim the help of that slippery creature, intuition. When an epiphany occurs, it leads us down new paths, gives us new passions to follow. Perhaps the most important thing we need for an epiphany to occur, however, is psychological preparedness for change. Otherwise it becomes too easy to close our eyes to new truths. To keep walking in the same comfortable groove, cosseted in the beliefs and conclusions that we hold to be so self-evident but are based more on opinion than fact.

***

Dr Jin Russell is on night shift on her first rotation as a paediatric registrar at Middlemore Hospital's emergency department. It is 2010. It's been a busy night. It is also freezing outside, in that cold, damp way that is peculiar to Auckland. The cold gets into your bones, and it definitely gets into your lungs, stirs up a legion of disease. There have been cases of croup and bronchiolitis to assess and treat – respiratory illnesses that always spike in winter. There's also been a few adolescent patients with alcohol intoxication, a child with pyelonephritis, a clutch of abdominal pains of various aetiologies.

Middlemore is the hospital for South Auckland, and its ED is the busiest in Australasia. Its catchment area is densely populated, and thus patients often present with diseases that are worsened by crowded living situations. The honey-crusted lesions of impetigo that leap from person to person. The unbearable itchiness of scabies, caused by a mite that burrows under the skin. Whooping cough, a highly contagious respiratory illness spread by coughing and sneezing, which can be fatal in babies younger than one year. Rheumatic fever, a disease entrenched in pockets in this country – not just South Auckland, but also in Northland and Waikato. No other developed country, other than Australia where Indigenous people are similarly afflicted, has such high rates of rheumatic fever. This disease, in which an untreated streptococcal infection of the throat can lead to an autoimmune reaction that damages heart valves, is directly linked to poverty and overcrowding. Ninety-five per cent of cases are Māori and Pasifika.

Jin sees five-year-old Bopha in ED that night. It is one in the morning, and the ED is still busy but settling down. The name Bopha translates as 'flower' in Cambodian. Bopha was born in New Zealand. Her parents were both born in Thai refugee camps after their own parents fled Cambodia during the turbulent 1970s regime of Pol Pot and the resulting genocide.

Tonight, Bopha is koala-hugging her father. The child has a delicate fall of fringe, brown eyes, a snub nose. She is shy but will smile at staff and puts up with being poked and prodded by them without too much fuss. She's used to these hospital visits; they happen all too often. An 'uncle' is also present, a family friend who is acting as an interpreter.

The child is a recurrent wheezer. She is tired, not just because of the hour of the night but also because she is working hard to breathe. She was wheezy all day, but got worse as the air temperature dropped overnight. Her dad tries to make her drink some juice, but she pushes his hand away. Jin can see Bopha's skinny ribs expanding and contracting under her thin night-shirt. Jin lifts the child's shirt to listen to her chest. The pocket of skin at the base of Bopha's neck sucks in, creating a circular depression, then blows out again. This is tracheal tug, indicating laboured breathing.

As part of a comprehensive medical history, Jin asks about the house the family lives in. The uncle says it is a rental that is crowded and cold. The family have asked a few times for better insulation, for a cleansing of the mould that runs like a constellation of black spores along some of the walls. The landlord has not been forthcoming. As immigrants with a tenuous grasp of English, the family find it hard to keep pushing for improvements to their living situation. Jin then asks where the mother is, presuming she is at home looking after the other kids. Instead, the uncle says: 'She's working. She's packing chickens in the factory.'

Jin walks back to her desk to write up the child's notes. When she sits down, however, she is incapable of writing. Her hands lie on the desk. She finds it hard to move past the fact that a mother cannot be with her sick child because she is packing chickens, to satisfy the edict that fresh food must be available as soon as supermarkets open. And that, in order to provide this, low-waged workers toil through the night, sometimes forgoing the needs of their loved ones.

Jin realises that, up till now, she's taken too much of this convenience for granted.

The nurse on call that night notices that Jin is on the verge of tears and quietly brings her a cup of tea and a biscuit as a small solace. They sit together for a while. Jin wonders if she would have been as upset if Bopha's mother had been working at the airport, selling cosmetics to travellers. She decides, on balance, that she probably wouldn't have been. There's something particularly hard about overnight factory work – the shifts that play havoc with circadian rhythms, the flicker of fluorescent lighting, the mindless repetitive tasks of wrap, box, stack, wrap, box, stack. The resulting exhaustion and sleep-deprivation.

Jin knows she is upset at the work the mother has to do, but also the multiple disadvantages that lead to this child's recurrent hospital visits. It's not just Bopha's asthma that is the issue. There's also the poor quality of the housing – condensation dripping down the windows, poorly insulated walls, mould on the ceilings, the overcrowding – all known risk factors for childhood illnesses. The fact that the family are migrants, with poor levels of English creating a greater risk of miscommunication and misunderstandings. The fragmented parental care. 'It struck me that we live in this society that allows the clustering of disadvantages to continue for some families, grossly affecting some children more than others.'

Bopha's mother arrives at 2 am, and the little girl clings to her like a limpet. Jin charts her regular salbutamol (an asthma-relieving medication) via a spacer (a clear plastic tube with a valve that connects to the inhaler, and improves asthma medicine getting into the lungs rather than hitting the back of the throat). Jin also checks if Bopha has a steroid inhaler as a preventer of further asthma attacks, and is using this regularly. She then admits her to the short-stay ward for observation overnight; she can probably go home in the morning. Jin is fairly certain, however, that Bopha will probably be back in a week or a month with the same issue.

The epiphany around the structural disadvantages that affect Bopha gets Jin thinking: what systemic factors influence health, positively or negatively? She has been reading *The Selfish Society* by Sue Gerhardt, with its tagline: 'How we all forgot to love one another and made money instead.' The premise is that more money and more 'stuff' does not make people happy. Rather, the pressures put on parents by modern society are detrimental to the health of children.

On another ED shift, she is on call with a colleague, who remarks, 'Look at this whiteboard. Croup, asthma, wheezing, skin infections, rheumatic fever. What is the single underlying disease for all these children? Poverty.'

Jin starts to focus on a different career trajectory for herself. 'At that point, I realised I could keep seeing individual children, treating them as best as I could and then sending them back to environments that were detrimental to their development, or I could dedicate myself to studying the health of populations, in order to analyse and hopefully change the systems that stratify people into pools of disadvantage.' Given her own life story, and her skills as a paediatrician, Jin believed she was well placed to pursue a path of advocacy and research alongside clinical medicine.

**

Ipoh, where Jin's parents grew up in the 1950s and 1960s, is the capital city of the Malaysian state of Perak. These days, it is known as the hipster capital of Malaysia. Its streets are clean, colonial-era British buildings dot the cityscape, and there is a vibrant food scene blending Chinese, Malay and Indian influences. There are limestone caves in the hills around the city, inside which Buddhist temples have been built; some of Jin's ancestors are buried at the feet of these caves.

Back in the 1970s, the rich tin deposits along the banks of the Kinta River ran out, and tin prices collapsed – thus the dynasty of Ipoh, which had seen this village boom into a city, was halted. Decades of decline set in before the more recent facelift brought the tourists back.

Jin's parents are ethnically Chinese: her mother's ancestors hail from Guangdong province in China, while her father's side is Hokkien, from Fujian province. They met at church as 11-year-olds, started 'going steady' in high school, and later, both went to medical school, but separately (Jin's father to the National University of Singapore, Jin's mother to the University of Malaya in Kuala Lumpur).

Wealth came and went in a boom–bust fashion for both of her parents' families. Jin's father was raised, alongside seven siblings, by his mother after her husband died; Jin's mother grew up wealthy for a time but money was lost along the way. Race riots that broke out in Kuala Lumpur in 1969 between ethnic Malay and Chinese left several hundred dead, and scarified the old wounds of racial distrust and tension, making them bleed afresh. The casualties were largely Chinese.

Jin's parents wanted something better. They flew to Christchurch in the mid-1970s and were overwhelmed by the beauty of the South Island, by the vastness of the Pacific Ocean overhung by moody skies, by the Southern Alps meandering like a snowy spine to the west of their new home city. Jin's brother was born, and later the family moved to Wellington, where Jin was born. Both siblings went to medical school in Auckland, completing the familial medical tetrad.

Matheson, Jin's husband, is an associate professor of philosophy at Auckland University. He is also a published author. In the Russells' home, there is one dead maidenhair fern sitting forlornly on the hallway table, but surrounding this unloved potplant are the writings of a variety of authors. Thomas Piketty's *Capital in the Twenty-first Century*. George Monbiot, Naomi Klein, Jeffrey Sachs.

Jin readily acknowledges that her own children are privy to a level of privilege that is vastly different from that of many of her young patients.

Her question became: how do disadvantage and deprivation affect a child's development?

In between her shifts, Jin interviewed paediatricians and other experts. She learnt that children behave differently growing up in a privileged home compared to growing up in a disadvantaged one. 'There's a noticeable contrast in different children's sense of agency,' she says. 'I remember putting in an intravenous line in a three-year-old child at Middlemore. I explained the process, and the mother said to the kid, "Be good for the doctor." So the kid just lay there, scared stiff, but compliant. Conversely, during a run at Starship ED in Auckland Hospital, I had to put in an intravenous line in a four-year-old boy. I explained the procedure to the mother, and she held the child in a bear hug and explained to him why he needed this thing to make him better. But he wasn't having a bar of it. He said loudly, over and over: "No, I don't want it, mummy, mummy, make it stop." At the age of four, this little boy had a much better sense of agency or control over his surroundings. He had a belief that his parent was powerful enough to stop bad things happening to him. This is not about culture, but about class. Children in certain circumstances can be conditioned to accept those in authority almost unquestioningly.'

She noticed gaps in expressive language as well, with children from affluent homes sometimes being almost two years ahead of their peers in terms of their vocabulary and reasoning. She remembered once asking a mother to read to her child to distract her. 'The mother opened the book slowly and said, "Okay, Mummy will read this to you, okay?" Then she proceeded to read hesitantly, with halting pauses. As she went on she started championing herself, saying, "I'm doing well!" and laughing out loud. She was enjoying reading a book to her daughter, and her daughter was mesmerised.'

When Jin began her research, there was an increasing amount of international data indicating that disadvantage and poverty were major determinants in stratifying children's health and educational outcomes. However, there was a significant lack of local data. The 'Growing Up in New Zealand' longitudinal study of children and families began in 2010 and Jin was invited to participate. The study is ongoing. It follows almost 7000 children (born 2009–2010) in the context of their families and the New Zealand environment, and helps inform policies to improve population well-being and reduce inequities in life-course outcomes.

Jin started a PhD in child epidemiology in 2013, specifically to study how disadvantage and poverty affect children's outcomes in the first five years of life. Previous research had cemented the link between disadvantage and a plethora of illnesses, but Jin's focus was broader and included the emotional and psychosocial sequelae of disadvantage. In the same way that wealth often begets more wealth, disadvantage can beget more disadvantage. Hence, illnesses and developmental setbacks can compound in the same child, leading to a Gestalt effect, where the whole is greater than the sum of the parts.

Focusing on the pre-school-age group, she analysed physical health and motor development, socio-emotional and behavioural functioning, and language, cognition and learning during three points in time: children aged nine months, two years, and four and a half years old. Using this data, she could then analyse the gaps between children from different backgrounds just before they entered school. What Jin found backed up international research. Essentially, children from more disadvantaged backgrounds had significantly worse outcomes in many of the areas mentioned above – physical health, behavioural function and learning – and the differences were evident as early as two years old. The question now became, what to do with this information?

There is an argument, which skitters back and forth across many societies, that each of us is responsible for the situation we find ourselves in. That, if people just worked harder, they'd flourish. That we are all given essentially the same opportunities in life. This argument is trotted out when it comes to discussing how much society should invest in the health and well-being of disadvantaged children. Surely, if the parents of these kids just stopped being so bloody lazy, got rid of the smokes and the booze and got themselves proper jobs, their children wouldn't need help from total strangers?

On the surface, there is some very superficial truth to this thinking. But scratch underneath and you'll find a whole host of factors that are not immediately apparent. Our physical, genetic and social milieux are strikingly different from one person to another. Children cannot choose where or when they are born, or how they are brought up. And sometimes, their parents are constrained by systemic factors.

Policymakers increasingly incorporate awareness of adverse childhood experiences (ACEs) into the way they approach children from disadvantaged backgrounds. ACEs are essentially toxic stress, and include illness, poverty, abuse, parents with mental-health issues and so on. Children exposed to ACEs have higher rates of depression, PTSD and suicide. They have higher rates of alcohol and drug use, and higher rates of teenage pregnancy leading to more premature delivery and foetal death. They end up with poorer educational opportunities and subsequent poor employment. They even have higher rates of chronic illness such as cancer and diabetes. Why does this not sound like a level playing field?

***

A child's brain is a soft, malleable organ, constantly developing and responding to its environment. Given the right circumstances, it is capable of incredible things. However, it is also incredibly sensitive to the physical, emotional and psycho-social soup around it. Positive, stable interaction with at least one caregiver is key to healthy development.

So, what's going on at a cellular and anatomic level in the brain of a child exposed to toxic stress? The key finding from many studies is that constant exposure to ACEs leads to a brain that is smaller in size and with a smaller surface area than the brain of a child who grows up in a healthy environment.[6] Research found that poverty alone, without any other types of toxic stress, can cause changes in children's brains. Bopha and children like her are susceptible to brain changes that can account for almost 20 per cent of the difference in their academic achievement when compared to peers from higher-income families. Studies in the USA have found that in the poorest families, income disparities of just a few thousand dollars are associated with major changes in brain structure. Cognitive skills, reading and memory all significantly declined with less parental income.[7] Yet, an increase in parental incomes between middle class and higher-income families led to much smaller gains in cognitive abilities in children. Thus, more money doesn't necessarily beget proportionately greater advantage.

Overall, it appears that a human child can learn to accommodate a wide variety of circumstances. Dropping slightly below median-income levels can be adapted to, but there is a point at which things topple off a cliff. In extreme poverty (which has knock-on effects on schooling, nutrition, sleep), the human brain seems to move out of the range of coping, and manifests life-long adverse sequelae.

Let's look at some of the structural changes in the brains of those who had childhood ACEs. MRI scans show that it's not just broken bones that we carry around with us, but invisibly changed brains that lead to visibly changed behaviour.[8] The hippocampus, for example, is involved in learning and memory, and also in regulating the stress hormone cortisol. With toxic stress, there may be a reduced hippocampal volume. Cortisol levels are either blunted or raised, depending on the level and type of stressor. This affects learning and socialisation, impairs the immune system, and increases the risk of affective (mood) disorders, such as anxiety and depression.

The corpus callosum is a thick bundle of nerve fibres, C-shaped in cross-section, that acts like high-speed broadband between the two halves of the brain, and helps with higher cognitive abilities, arousal and emotion; it, too, may be shrunken in size. The cerebellum is a striated walnut-shaped bit of the brain that sits underneath the larger cerebral hemispheres, and is situated near the nape of the neck. It is often underdeveloped in children exposed to ACEs. Good cerebellar function is vital for coordinating motor behaviour and executive function.

Those who were severely neglected as children often have smaller prefrontal cortices in their teens and adulthood – this part of the brain helps with emotional regulation and behaviour. The prefrontal cortex sits at the front of the brain. In the not-so-distant past, it was intentionally severed during the now-discredited neurosurgical procedure known as a frontal lobotomy.

Abuse and neglect doesn't seem to change the size of the amygdala in the brain, but it does change its function, leading to a state of hyperarousal, a constant fight-or-flight activation, and an ongoing meerkat-like vigilance of surroundings.

Burrow deeper still and look at DNA, those intertwining double helices that are the blueprint of almost all life on Planet Earth. What happens to these molecular strands that hold our unique genetic codes when they are exposed to chronic stress?

Epigenetic studies have found that DNA itself may not be altered by chronic stress, but the expression of our genes can be.[9] Chemical markers attach themselves to various bits of our DNA, to turn them on or off depending on exposure to a positive or negative environment. Specifically, those exposed to toxic stress showed changes in the expression of the serotonin transporter gene. This then led to increased threat-related amygdala reactivity. The study's authors found that greater amygdala reactivity was linked to later depressive symptoms.

There is some evidence that epigenetic changes can be transmitted down through the generations – the things that we may carry with us from our mothers' wombs. Other studies have also shown that telomeres can be shortened by chronic stress.[10] Our DNA is arranged into chromosomes inside our cells, and the telomeres are like tiny caps sitting at the end of DNA to stop them fraying too early. You could compare telomeres to the plastic protective tips at the ends of shoelaces. Telomeres naturally shorten with age, and thus send signals to ageing cells to stop dividing. Grow old now, they say. However, this natural shortening is speeded up in the presence of chronic stress; thus telomeres are used by scientists as a proxy biological marker for chronic stress.

Multiple studies have found that telomere length is shortened in adults in a variety of stressful situations: poverty, mental illness (particularly depression), domestic violence, smoking, obesity. Shortened telomere length is associated with higher rates of age-related disease such as cancer and heart disease, and earlier mortality. It's like chronic stress 'weathers' people, reducing their resilience and making them more susceptible to the curveballs that life may throw at them. Conversely, a positive environment – a good diet, a safe family home, a healthy community – can reduce the rate at which telomeres shorten.

So what does a child with these changes in brain function, anatomy, genetics and neurochemical activity look or act like? Children with these changes show a constant fear response and hyperarousal, even in situations that are not threatening. They may lose the ability to differentiate between danger and safety. This generalised fear response can lead in later life to a greater incidence of anxiety and post-traumatic stress disorder. Their fear response can be triggered too easily by eye contact, by a simple touch on the arm – non-threatening actions that may be misinterpreted. Because they are constantly monitoring their environments for threatening non-verbal cues, they are less able to interpret and respond to verbal cues, even in a typically safe environment such as a classroom, which means they are unable to be calm enough to learn properly, and may be labelled as learning disabled.

Child maltreatment may permanently alter areas of the brain involved in emotion and stress regulation. This can be seen in adulthood: those who respond poorly to stressful situations, such as medical illness or job loss, almost invariably have had a stressful childhood. Good connectivity between the amygdala and the hippocampus may be lost, leading to the development of anxiety and depression, even as early as adolescence. Early emotional abuse or severe deprivation can also alter the brain's ability to use serotonin, the key neurotransmitter that stabilises our mood and creates feelings of well-being and happiness, as well as helping with sleeping, eating and digestion.

These children may have diminished executive functioning. Good executive functioning of our brains requires three components: a good working memory; inhibitory control to filter out thoughts and impulses; and mental flexibility so that we can adapt to change. It helps us to achieve academic and career success, and improves everyday social interactions. Toxic stress can cause a reduction in executive functioning even from an early age. Such children are less able to filter out unnecessary thoughts, manage multiple ideas or have a good working memory. They may have a weakened response to positive feedback, and they may also react incorrectly in social situations (for example, misreading a peer's neutral face as aggressive). The brain alterations caused by toxic stress can result in lower IQ and lower academic achievement.[11]

It's not just a failure to meet a child's physical needs for food, safety and shelter that causes stress to that child. It can also be a failure to meet their cognitive, emotional and social needs. Children need support and encouragement from their caregivers in order to thrive; failure in this regard leads to delayed developmental milestones such as language acquisition, cognition and physical prowess.

Sobering, isn't it?

***

In 1855, the American abolitionist and author Frederick Douglass, in dialogue with white slave owners about the perpetuating effects of slavery, wrote: 'It is easier to build strong children than to repair broken men.'

The drive to help all children flourish and reach their full potential is a very personal one for Dr Jin Russell. She believes her mum's older sister in Malaysia had rheumatic fever. This aunt had a childhood illness where she could not walk; as an adult she was easily fatigued. She had open heart surgery in her fifties and was put on warfarin. Due to mismanagement of this anticoagulation, she suffered a massive stroke, developed dementia and died in her sixties. 'Malaysia was a third-world country back then, and illnesses like rheumatic fever were rife. Imagine my parents' surprise, then, on coming to New Zealand and working as doctors here, to find these same diseases rampant in the underclass of New Zealand. Why is this? It is like part of New Zealand got left behind.'

It is not possible to remove all forms of disadvantage. There will always be circumstance, mental-health issues, sudden redundancies or ill health to deal with. But certain things can be changed. The most important thing, Jin believes, is to 'decluster disadvantage'. To stop the domino effect where one bad thing leads to another which leads to yet another. Children like Bopha can't be expected to cope with income poverty, poor housing, parental mental-health issues, parents working long hours or doing shift work, and other disadvantages all at the same time, and still thrive.

Poverty is the most fundamental thing that needs to be addressed, as it affects so many other things. It's not just a question of social policy. It's a biomedical problem, an environmental condition that affects some children more than others. Different people respond to the same stressors in physiologically different ways, depending on their genetic heritage and their social milieu. Some studies have found that improving a family's income can lead to an improvement in a child's cognitive and language skills within 18 months to two years.

Prevention is key. Efforts for at-risk families should focus on protective factors that help strengthen families, prevent abuse and neglect, and promote healthy brain development. These efforts may help prevent normal adverse events from becoming ongoing toxic stress. Such efforts include concrete financial and social support for parents. It includes building up parental resilience and improving parental skills. It's important to provide an environment for a child that is nurturing, stable, predictable, understandable and supportive.

'The goal of paediatric care is to maximise each child's potential,' Jin says. 'This is something that we should all be striving for. After all, these children are our future citizens, our future workers, our future champions of resilient societies.'

The greatness and pain that our ancestors gave

patient: Arama*; GP: Dr Himali McInnes

If there is one patient who has opened my eyes to my own cognitive bias and who has helped me to recognise the profound effect of the past on a person's health, it is my patient Arama*.

'Hey, what's up, doc?' says Arama as he walks into my consulting room one day. He's weaving a little, his breath reeks of alcohol, his speech is slurred. He wants to get some antibiotics for a chesty cough that he's had for a week.

It's 10 am on a busy Monday morning. My consulting room in Māngere, South Auckland, is spacious, full of light. The view outside is of the large Māngere shopping centre carpark. I've stuck up colourful posters on the walls, some medical, some deliberately non-medical; my favourite is a print of New Zealand birds that I bought at Te Papa – a cromolithograph (c. 1900) by William Schmidt, based on Walter Buller's *A History of the Birds of New Zealand.*

I've known Arama for years. He's a Māori patient in his fifties and he has the chronic lung condition bronchiectasis. He is a life-long smoker, with multiple attempts to quit under his belt and, as I have recently discovered, he also drinks excessively at times. He and his partner are living in someone's cold, draughty garage. Over the course of a decade, I have doled out multiple antibiotic scripts for Arama's illness-prone lungs. Each time, I ask him to stop smoking. We discuss using community services to help him reduce his intake of alcohol. He tries, off and on, but finds it hard to engage with them. I write letters to Housing New Zealand pleading his case – a patient with a chronic lung condition needs better accommodation than a cold garage – but the answer is always the same. Too many people needing a home, not enough houses. I try to organise insulation for his current residence, but find out that he doesn't qualify for this.

Arama seems to take on board my advice every now and then, but usually he slips back into old habits. And so he keeps turning up to my room with his cough: a symphony of wheeze, productive of purulent green sputum, oleaginous gunk that plugs his airways and curtails his potential.

When Arama is sober, he is funny, self-deprecating, smart-mouthed. We laugh lots together. He has a savvy street-smart intelligence, an appraising air. He follows complex medical logic better than other patients. He struggles with his addictions; he doesn't want them, yet he keeps coming back to them. He has aspirations for a better life, just like anyone else, but the hole he is in is particularly large and particularly difficult to get out of. His inability to change causes me immense frustration for several years. I know objectively that there are certain measures that can help this patient, so why won't he just take my advice? Aren't some of the changes he needs to make simple enough to do?

***

I clearly remember the revelation on this particular Monday morning that changes my understanding and my attitude towards Arama. He's in a talkative mood, and we get to chatting about this and that. Maybe the alcohol has loosened his tongue and lowered his defences. At any rate, he lets slip an off-hand comment: 'Yeah, I got a lot of shit growing up. I was molested, eh.'

I sit back and look at him. The birds on the Te Papa print above my desk – the tūī, the blue-helmeted thuggery of kōtare, the wise but sleepy ruru – still their rustling and preening as they listen. I'd been so stuck in my medical frame of mind, diagnosing and fixing Arama's physical complaints, that I hadn't taken enough notice of his 'iceberg'. That submerged clod of memories, experiences and beliefs we drag around with us, that we rarely show to others, that we may in fact be unaware of. The things we carry from our childhood. The thumbprints of our ancestors on our souls.

A patient rarely presents with their iceberg, but it affects their health in multiple ways and can be more important than the presenting complaint. Yet there's a stigma to disclosing past abuse or addictions. Or the fact that a social situation is unsafe, riddled with violence, beset by vulnerability. It's too hard to divulge emotional pain, easier to talk about physical pain.

This conversation with Arama happens at about the same time that I'm reading up on New Zealand history. All that 'forgotten' history. I'd lived in New Zealand for 25 years by this stage, yet this was the first time I was finding out about these events – the land confiscations, the killing of unarmed men, women and children, the smothering of a language. The justifications for violence, the grossly unequal wars that were fought on trumped-up charges. The fact that many sites of historical significance are hardly signposted, even today.

My reading had made me start to think about the generational ramifications of trauma on health. How much of an impact does land loss and loss of culture have on the health of individuals alive today? What are the ongoing effects on the colonisers themselves, and on more recent arrivals like myself? Some might say there is no impact – let the past be the past, let's focus on the here and now, let's stop making excuses. Others might say that the past provides a resounding explanation for ongoing disparities in health and other outcomes. The problem with the past is that it is invisible, too easy to dismiss.

Certainly it appears Māori have not forgotten New Zealand's disruptive history of colonisation. European New Zealanders were also escapees of brutal systems in their countries of origin: the class hierarchy of England, the famines of Ireland, the burning fires of the Scottish Highlands. Yet, in New Zealand, the insatiable hunger for new land caused a repetition of the same sorts of oppression that the new settlers had ostensibly left behind.

When Arama starts to describe his childhood, I am in a receptive frame of mind. The next patient will have to wait. Over the course of today's consultation, and further consults later on, I learn a lot about Arama. I start to recognise that he does not exist in isolation to the things that have come before, or the things around him now. His health and well-being are inextricably influenced by his childhood, which in turn is influenced by the lives of his parents, and their parents before them.

He tells me that he was adopted by extended whānau, in a practice known as whāngai. 'I was the youngest in the family, and quickly became Dad's pet. This made my older adopted brothers and sisters jealous. Even now, there is still ill feeling – all these years later.'

Arama's adoptive father worked as a truck driver; his adoptive mother was a seasonal orchard worker, and she spoke te reo Māori, 'But she never shared this with us, Doc, cos she was strapped for speaking it.' His father had fought in World War II, but he did not talk of his experiences. 'I wish he'd shared some of that stuff. I think it really scarred him for life, eh.' After returning from the war, Māori ex-servicemen were sometimes left to fend for themselves. The assumption was that they would have access to tribal land – an incorrect assumption, as less than 10 per cent of land remained in Māori ownership by then.[12]

***

Dr Len Prior*, whom I write about in another chapter, has a different narrative. His Pākehā ex-serviceman father received a rehabilitation loan, bought land, owned his own house. Len's dad developed alcoholism due to presumed post-traumatic stress disorder, the awful legacy of 'shellshock'. However, Len's mother was able to keep working and provide for her kids because they had their own home. Perhaps owning land and a house would have given Arama's adoptive father a much better shot at life. As it was, he became a heavy drinker; Arama believes now that he had PTSD.

Arama says of himself, 'I was quite bright when I was young.' He remembers enjoying school as a child. The extended family was large, with lots of relatives who came and went. His mother's family were reasonably well educated, but poor. Arama remembers a childhood devoid of opulence or treats, but he felt loved, especially by his father.

There was always alcohol in the house, thanks to his father's alcoholism, and parties were a common occurrence. It was at times a chaotic place to be a child. Arama started to get sexually abused by various male relatives from the age of six onwards – an uncle, some cousins. When Arama was 11, his adoptive mother died of a sudden bleed in the brain at just 48. It triggered a marked worsening in Arama's fortunes: his adoptive father, wracked by grief, left the kids in the care of extended family and went trucking for months at a time.

Bereft of both his parents, Arama started to drink – he'd already started smoking at the age of nine. When he was about 14, he remembers getting a severe bout of pneumonia and not getting treated. I suspect this paved the way for his bronchiectasis. After leaving school, he got a job at a factory. However, he started to drink heavily, with almost daily marijuana use. 'I went through a bad patch from 18 onwards. It's like I saw it, so I did it. I felt like I had it all, friends, booze, parties, but actually I think I was mentally unstable, feeling abandoned by Dad. So I drank and drank.'

Stints in various jobs followed, but most didn't last long as he got swayed by 'girls and parties'. He tried to do some courses, including learning te reo Māori, but found studying was hard as an adult despite having enjoyed it as a child. He failed all his courses. 'I felt like I was not spiritually or mentally sound enough to learn my own language.'

Arama met his long-term partner in the early 2000s. She is ten years older. Theirs has been a fractious relationship. Recently, she was assaulted by an acquaintance and suffered a traumatic brain injury, so Arama is now her full-time carer. He thinks about leaving her often, but guilt makes him stay. At any rate, he is unable to afford a place on his own.

We finish our chat. I'm running 30 minutes late, but I've learnt a whole lot more about my patient than I could have during a doctor-led consult.

***

A little bit about my own background, and how privilege can be traced back to the actions of our ancestors, in the same way Arama's story has its roots in the past. I was born in Sri Lanka, but left there at the age of one when my parents headed to Malaysia. It was the 1970s. Sri Lanka was teetering on the edge of socialist chaos, despite possessing great natural wealth and sublime tourist-luring beauty. This was in part a colonial legacy bestowed by the British, who encouraged tea and rubber plantations at the expense of rice and food. Morale was low, inflation and internal dissension were high. So my parents left for the bright lights of Petaling Jaya and then, later, Kuala Lumpur.

As an adult pondering the vagaries of privilege and good fortune, I would later pinpoint this migration as a pivotal moment. The Malaysian economy was starting to pick up pace in the 1970s as it transitioned from mining and agriculture to multiple other industries. My parents were highly sought after middle-class professionals: my father was an accountant, my mother, a doctor. Meanwhile, my cousins who stayed behind in Sri Lanka suffered through school and university closures due to bomb threats during a 26-year civil war, and consequently, most of them did not pursue tertiary education, despite possessing

121

robust intellectual acumen. Hence, in the space of just one generation, different choices and outcomes became available to people of the same genetic potential.

We tried to settle back in Sri Lanka for a few years. We built a house, we thought we'd make it work, but there was unrest and suspicion floating on the wind. The genesis of Sri Lanka's civil war, the killing of 13 Sinhala policemen by Tamil separatists in the northern town of Jaffna, occurred in 1983. This led to race riots and the massacre of approximately 3000 innocent Tamil civilians, so my family fled again, this time to Papua New Guinea. Contracts for expats were good. I went to an international school that I remember with great fondness.

After high school, my parents wanted to send my brother and me to a good university. We considered Australia but I was relieved when we chose New Zealand instead. I didn't want to go to the 'lucky but racist country'. My 15-year-old self had this impression of New Zealand as a land of equality and fairness, an egalitarian island rippling with forests and cool mountains, where the indigenous Māori had made great strides compared to other colonised peoples around the world. No one took particular pains to dispel this notion, not even when I went through the citizenship ceremony years later.

I'd always wanted to be a vet, but then decided I'd be a doctor and keep pets on the side. Also, I had vague notions of helping people. It's funny how poorly one's impression of a life in medicine tallies with reality. Once we hit the hospitals as junior house surgeons, we were so green it was frightening. We literally held power over life and death. We could alter someone's existence with a slash of our pens, yet photos from that time show me so achingly fresh-faced. 'When is the doctor coming?' patients would ask me.

There was a vivid perception among many of us that Māori patients were 'difficult'. 'Why do people have to be hostile right from the start?' I remember thinking. 'Why this chip on the shoulder?' I was just trying to do my job.

All of this happened so long ago. Twenty years ago. Were those patients actually hostile or were they simply unwell? Were they acting defensively because of previous poor medical treatment? Were there in fact many Māori patients who were perfectly lovely to deal with, but I only noticed those who fitted my preconceived bias? I am not sure. I do know, though, that my understanding of Māori culture and society only extended to a *Once Were Warriors* stereotype. All that alcohol, the domestic violence, the gang culture, the drugs. It seemed clear to me that this was a lifestyle choice made by some Māori, and that they only had themselves to blame. We learnt about the Treaty of Waitangi and basic race relations as part of our ongoing medical training, but even that did little to dispel my skewed perceptions.

Luckily, it's possible for a place to open your eyes. South Auckland did that for me. I started as a general practitioner there in 2009. It gave me a valuable insight into just how tough life can be for some New Zealanders. Despite all the hardship, South Auckland thrums with kindness and gratitude. People stop their vehicles to let you cross the road when there is no pedestrian crossing; children are cherished; the elderly are looked after by teenagers; sweet grandmas kiss you noisily on the cheek as they thank you.

South Auckland taught me that there is a huge difference in the choices (educational, economic, health-related) available to children when they are growing up, and these differences continue into adulthood. Warren Buffett, the American business tycoon and philanthropist, recognises that he 'won the ovarian lottery' by being born white and male in America. I won my own ovarian lottery by being born to middle-class, well-educated South Asian parents who had the freedom to emigrate where they wished.

It took South Auckland to switch me from thinking individually to thinking communally. Back in 2016, as the housing crisis deepened, a lot of my patients resorted to sleeping in their cars. Rents had risen steeply, and house prices were outstripping incomes. I started seeing many patients with rattly chests and laboured breathing. Physical repercussions of economic deprivation. Around that time, a friend gave me a book to read: *Pākehā and the Treaty: Why it's our Treaty too* by Patrick Snedden. I became aware of a morass of history that cast a very different light on this supposedly fair and egalitarian country. Vincent O'Malley's *The Great War for New Zealand* is comprehensive in its documentation of how the Waikato Land Wars shaped this nation. Prior to the confiscation of their land, many Māori had incorporated European farming methods. Fruit trees blossomed with the scent of honey. Flour was milled for bread. Sheep and cattle were reared and sold. Rangiaowhia was the 'breadbasket of the Waikato'. When the British Army torched the lot in February 1864, it precipitated economic collapse among the southern Waikato tribes.

How do you stay healthy when you lose your livelihood and your land? I started to see the chain of events that helped explain some of Arama's current situation. We didn't learn about New Zealand history in medical school. Yet the legacy of what has happened in the past still persists. It has an impact on the health of Māori men, women and children living today.

***

The World Health Organization has described colonisation as *the* most significant social determinant of health affecting Indigenous people worldwide. The fact that the effects of colonisation are somewhat invisible today leads to denial and persistent arguments against its relevance. It is frustrating.

Pre-European-contact Māori possibly had life expectancies similar to Europeans of the time, but the introduction of European diseases into an immunologically naive population led to a rapid decline in numbers. The land wars and land confiscation led to further decline in health and population numbers through malnutrition and reduced economic well-being. By the 1880s, Māori life expectancy fell as low as the mid-twenties, and the population dropped from about 100,000 to about 42,000 people.

A new generation of Māori leaders arose in the 1890s. Apirana Ngata and others advocated for Māori development of the land that remained under Māori ownership (30 per cent) in order to improve sanitation and nutrition. These measures helped raise the population to 100,870 by the end of World War II. However, Māori land ownership by this time was just 10 per cent, and although gains in life expectancy were made, the disparity with Pākehā was still 15 years.

Before World War II, more than 80 per cent of Māori lived in rural areas. After the war, tangata whenua, especially the younger generation, migrated en masse to the cities, looking for employment in urban industries. It was a big shift, both in terms of location and in terms of culture. There was a severance with the whenua and with whānau, and it led to significant health and socioeconomic sequelae. Some Māori flourished in the new circumstances; others did not. Loneliness and unemployment morphed into antisocial behaviour for some. This is the social schism later depicted in Alan Duff's *Once Were Warriors*, and it became the dominant stereotype of Māori for me and others.

The twentieth century saw a 'Māori renaissance'; an acknowledgement that, far from being a dying race, this was a people that was on the rise politically, culturally and artistically. In terms of health, there's been steady improvements in life expectancy, although the discrepancy is still around seven years. Tuberculosis has been virtually eradicated. Healthier lifestyles have been adopted. Childhood mortality has dropped. Yet significant disparities in health outcomes and access still exist. Why?

Chimamanda Ngozi Adichie, in a TED talk titled 'The danger of the single story', warns how limited contact with a group of people can lead to stereotypes, allow prejudices to take root and perpetuate discriminatory behaviours. I don't want Arama's story to represent this singular narrative. I'm grateful that he has been brave enough to share his story. He wants it out there: he's thrilled that someone has written about him. He wants acknowledgement of the shit that happened in his childhood, because it's not fair or right that such things should happen to a child. But his story is more complex than just endless bad stuff. He's a survivor, and I admire his grit. What allows some people to flourish while others flounder?

Different people respond differently to various life situations, depending on their genetic and biological constitution as well as environmental factors. However, it appears that for many who have done well, regardless of ethnicity or background, there are some factors working in their favour. In particular, people do well when they get help and support from at least one other person.

Consider a Māori man at my church who had been in prison for a violent crime for 13 years. By the time he was released, he was a changed man. He helped out as a volunteer in the church kitchen for two years, and worked hard and without complaint. He was there early to set up, he stayed late to do the dishes. He was utterly trustworthy with the petty cash. For two years he was on the unemployment benefit. He went to scores of job interviews but kept getting turned down. He was a brown man in his fifties with a prison record. In the meantime, another ex-prisoner, this time a Pākehā man, who was a decade older and who had been in prison for 12 years for a sex crime, also came to our church. He found a job within months.

The Māori man became depressed with his lack of success in getting a job. He told me, 'I may as well go back to prison, Himali, because there's nothing for me out here.' I asked him where his current job interview was. I then secretly contacted that workplace, writing a letter that outlined this man's work ethic and trustworthiness. I wrote how, so far, no one had given him a chance. I used the clout of my 'doctor' title to sign off the letter. He got that job and he's now still in employment, has bought his own car and is renting a place from his own income.

Although the disadvantages faced by Māori due to overcrowding and poor access to healthcare improved in the latter half of the twentieth century, significantly poorer health outcomes still exist today.[13] A plethora of factors are at play: sub-standard housing, poorer education, cultural alienation, land loss, lower incomes and discrimination. A number of initiatives, such as VLCA (very low cost access) health practices have been set up to try to reduce barriers. There is extra funding for Māori and Pasifika patients. Dental care is free for children till age 18. There are some iwi-based health trusts who are looking into new and innovative methods of providing culturally resonant care to address inequities.

Yet disparities still exist. Reducing the cost of consults only improves one barrier. Patients with low-paying jobs often can't afford to take time off to go to the doctor. There is also inequitable behaviour by health practitioners. I know all too well that institutional racism or, at the very least, institutional bias, occurs. I harboured it myself, I am ashamed to admit, back when I believed that all of us are wholly responsible for the situations we find ourselves in, without understanding the wider societal, familial and historical contexts that affect us all.

Here's a verbatim transcript of a letter written to a GP colleague by a hospital specialist about a Māori patient in 2019:

> Going forward, management of his COPD [chronic obstructive pulmonary disease] would usually include a referral to pulmonary rehabilitation but I think he is unlikely to attend this due to his social set-up. He would never be a candidate for a bullectomy, lung transplant, or lung volume reduction surgery, and sadly I think his health is going to catch up with him in his poor social circumstances. Otherwise I am afraid that I have little else that we can offer him, and I hope that his social situation improves so that he can try and focus on his health. No further clinic review has been arranged. Yours sincerely ...

This letter spelt the end of that patient's accessible healthcare. He now has terminal lung cancer. No patient should be declined healthcare on the basis of their challenging or dysfunctional social situation. Improving the health outcomes for disadvantaged groups, which includes disadvantaged Pākehā, Pasifika peoples and immigrants, needs to encompass a whole-of-society approach.

It's the fundamental right of every person to be able to flourish, to reach their full potential.

The saying goes that addiction does not discriminate. That it doesn't give a shit about who it leaves howling with pain, drowning in shallow water, clinging to a cliff face. The truth is, addiction does discriminate. It's much more likely to afflict people who have been scarred by trauma. Thanks to improved funding for mental healthcare for Māori and Pasifika patients, Arama is able to access a trained psychologist at no cost. He is slowly unravelling the effects of his ancestral and childhood legacies on his current health.

'If I could go back and change things, Doc, I'd definitely get rid of the people who abused me. They'd be the first ones I'd shoot!' he says, laughing ruefully.

It's likely that Arama's teenage pneumonia led to his chronic bronchiectasis. This impacts on his ability to study or work because of poor energy levels. His social situation is also hard to break out of without help. Yet he acknowledges a degree of responsibility. 'The counsellor helped me recognise factors that were out of my control when I was a child. I've now got to take responsibility for some things I do – the smoking, the drinking – and own it. But, Doc, it's hard. I still feel like my whole being is being criticised all the time. It's hard to break that kōrero. But I want to get better.'

***

For myself, every time a patient comes into my consulting room these days, I try to be aware of the hidden things that float in their wake: the threads of history twining through their flesh, the invisible strands that wield so much influence on their health and behaviour. And I try to be aware, as much as possible, of the biases that press shut my eyes and my ears to someone else's truth.

Meth, manslaughter and mercy

prisoner: Jade*; trauma therapist: Catarina*
Jade's story is a composite of real narratives, for purposes of
confidentiality.

'You stay, here Jade*! Use this knife if you have to.' Matt* shoves a knife into Jade's hands. It's an old kitchen knife, the blade whetted against a stone so many times it sings with sharpness. He points to the bathroom. Jade stumbles in, still wearing the jeans and sweatshirt she's been wearing all night. There's only a small high window in the bathroom; she should be safe in there. Matt picks up a loaded gun as he slips outside.

***

A party with some of their mates had finished late. There'd been joints of marijuana. They'd passed around a bong, smoked crystals of methamphetamine. It's now three in the morning but neither Matt nor Jade feel sleepy; instead, they feel wired. They talk and talk, and sometimes they snap at each other in irritation. There's a flood of dopamine in their systems released by the meth, and they feel on top of the world. The short-term pleasure of meth is so strong, it's hard to consider the long-term terror of it.

The frenzied barking of their dogs alerts them to intruders. Matt springs to the window and looks out, past the shipping container plonked in the yard – the metal box a deliberate ploy to screen the house from prying passers-by. The boundary fence is tall with a strip of carpet tack running along the top edge. Sharp enough to shred fingers.

Moonlight floods the garden of their Wairarapa home. Matt can see at least three or four shadowy figures prowling the perimeter of the property. He can't clearly see their faces, but by their bulk and stealth, he's sure these are members of a rival gang, probably on the hunt for weapons and drugs. There's plenty of both in the house. Like milk and bread, they are staples in this gang pad.

Matt lets the dogs out of their kennels and they rush towards the fence, growling and snapping. Matt follows, his senses wired, the gun a cold shadow in his hand.

From inside, Jade can hear shouting and cursing. She stays still. Her head pounds like a drum from the swirl of alcohol and meth. She needs to pee but adrenaline also pumps through her. 'Stupid arseholes', she thinks, 'trying to get our stash of ice. Bastards.'

'F-ark!' someone yells from the garden. There's a thud, the sound of wood splitting, and then a scuffle. The front door slams open and somebody stumbles inside.

Jade grips her knife. Through the crack in the bathroom door, she can hear someone crashing into things in the living room. She's pumped. She's furious. Her teeth clench, she licks her dry, cracked lips. She's sure she's about to be attacked. She thinks she hears a voice: 'I'm gonna get you good, bitch.' She pushes the door open. Jumps on the shadowy figure in the living room, stabs with the knife. There's the satisfying feel of metal sliding between ribs, slicing warm flesh. 'Just like sticking a pig,' she thinks. No sweat.

Some time later – is it minutes or hours? – she turns the light on. Matt is lying in a pool of blood. Jade screams in terror. She scoops him up in her arms and yells at him to wake up. The police arrive, followed by an ambulance.

Matt doesn't wake up.

***

Trauma therapist Catarina* meets Jade shortly after she comes into prison. To this day, Jade's story is hard to forget. It's such a shocking thing, to kill your own partner. Jade's story reminds Catarina of the trauma in her own past.

Normally, there is a long waiting list to see Catarina. Jade gets bumped to the top because of the enormity of her grief, the severity of her crime. Catarina's job is to assess her physical safety initially, as Jade is at high risk of self-harming.

Jade's pain is so acute, so visceral, it bubbles out of her eyes in salty tears, torrents out of her mouth in an unending wail. She's in her twenties, her skin peppered with a bloom of acne, a streak of defiant pink curling through her hair. She kicks and flails against the custodial staff in an anger so fierce she is like a caged animal. The staff are trained to be equanimous, impermeable in the face of such eruptive behaviour. Jade is placed in the ISU (Intervention and Support Unit) for safety. Prisoners in ISU are deemed to be at risk of self-harm, so are checked on every 15 minutes. There is no privacy for showers or ablutions, again, because of the risk of self-harming.

Catarina teases out the threads of Jade's story. Jade remembers a lack of boundaries for herself and her siblings while growing up. Her freewheeling Māori mother was little more than a child herself, the product of a broken home, squeezed through the mill of multiple foster families. Jade's Pākehā father disappeared early on, and she's had no contact with him. Her mum often referred to Jade's father as scum, as a loser who couldn't hold down a job because he was too busy drinking.

There were numerous 'uncles' in the house. These were not kind or jovial men, and in fact were not even relatives – but they were perpetrators of pain to a young Jade and her siblings, under the sheets of her childhood bed, in the place where a child should feel safe. And after one such uncle pulled her by her hair and kicked her out of the house after an argument, 12-year-old Jade ran away. She ended up under a Wellington bridge, and prostituted herself in order to buy food, alcohol, cigarettes. She fell for a boy.

Matt was living rough also. Jade remembers how she fell in love with his eyes first. Green in some lights, grey in others, flecked with gold like two distant suns. Matt's father was an alcoholic who thrashed his children, so Matt ran away from home. He was just 13 at the time. Jade and Matt banded together for safety with some other street kids; the girls were easy targets for older men and it was safer to be in a group. Everyone dabbled in meth and marijuana. 'I was so fucked up with pain on the inside,' Jade tells Catarina. 'The drugs just took it all away.' Jade and Matt fell in with a local gang near Wellington. They were both still kids. The paper chain that was their lives was easily torn. The gang promised to be family. Matt got bashed a couple of times as a new prospect, but he passed the induction. Jade was passed around some of the older gang members. She put up with it; longer term, she knew there'd be the security of gang protection and a good supply of the meth she was rapidly becoming dependent on. Jade still remembers the first time she tried meth. The rush she got from it. After just that one time, she was hooked, desperate for more.

Even though she knew it was cut with all sorts of stuff – paint thinner, battery acid, drain cleaner, antifreeze – and even though it was disintegrating the substance of her flesh, she couldn't get enough of it. Now, all Jade has are the gun-grey walls of a prison cell and Matt, the love she'd hoped to grow old with, is gone. This is Jade's first time in prison. She will be convicted of manslaughter.

***

Catarina is open-faced and friendly. Her blue eyes are warm; she is frequently tactile. Her smile is comforting. Beneath the softness, however, there is steel and a fierce determination to make a difference in the lives of traumatised women.

Catarina was born in New Zealand. When she was two years old, her mother took her and her older brother and returned to Europe. Home life was turbulent, violent, but in the midst of it all was Catarina's grandmother, Oma, the one person who provided an anchor, who made a difference. Oma was a wise, straight-up woman who'd lived through two world wars. Her psyche was shaped by grit, grenades and scarcity. 'She was generous,' Catarina recalls. 'She gave intelligently, not foolishly. She was good at saying no when she needed to – an important lesson for me to learn.'

Oma encouraged Catarina to write and make art whenever she felt sad or unmoored, to trace out her thoughts in pencil and paper, paint and ink. Catarina credits Oma for her life-long love of learning, her desire to help other people. She also relished the cathartic power of art. Coloured pencils, charcoal, graphite – mute sticks that helped her articulate difficult emotions. She attended art school with the intention of teaching art, but one day while visiting a patient in a mental institution, she had an insight. It was like 'lightning from heaven' she says. 'I realised that I actually hated the pretentiousness of the arts scene. I loved art – I still do – but not all the garbage that went with it. And sitting there in that mental-health hospital, I looked around and all I could see were charts full of medicines, and patients that seemed only half alive. I thought, "I want to be an art therapist." I want to help people heal with colour and feeling.'

Around this time, Catarina fell into a deep depression. Her traumatic childhood was bubbling up, festering like a sore. She contacted her father and flew back to New Zealand to be with him. She married and had children. She completed a diploma in visual arts, majored in sculpture ceramics. Then she enrolled at Whitecliffe, New Zealand's first arts-therapy school, completing a master's in clinical arts therapy. She learnt how to guide clients to use their creativity to bring emotional, physical, spiritual and mental well-being to their lives. She also completed a postgraduate diploma in counselling and guidance, and then started work as a prison trauma therapist.

'Everyone has some trauma in their lives,' Catarina says. 'All trauma counsellors need to attempt therapy for themselves first. Significant trauma needs intervention to prevent longer-term PTSD.'

When Catarina came back to New Zealand in the 1980s, race issues were becoming more prominent in the national consciousness. All through her training, Catarina learnt of Treaty issues, of the effects of colonisation. As a New Zealander with a strong European accent, Catarina has herself been the target of hurtful and disparaging racist remarks. Her former husband, a Pākehā New Zealander, was unable to access scholarships in medical training while other students with lower grades could. This still rankles her. 'However, I don't align myself with black or white issues. This is why prisoners tend to trust me. They have "eyes in their gut", they know if you are prejudiced. The reason they are in prison is of secondary importance to me. The core issue for me regarding the girls in prison is their human dignity and how to restore it.'

Last Christmas, Catarina went in on her own time to visit 'the girls'. Special occasions like Christmas are incredibly hard for prisoners, so she took along kindness and a listening ear. One more step in the process of restoring dignity and hope.

***

As of June 2020, according to the Department of Corrections, there were almost 9000 men in prison in New Zealand. Female prisoners numbered nearly 600. Roughly one-third of these prisoners were on remand, awaiting trial or sentencing. More than one-third were affiliated with gangs. There were a further 28,000 people serving their sentences under community orders. There are 18 prisons in New Zealand, including one private one. Three of these prisons house female prisoners. There are additionally four youth-justice residencies. Some of our prisons are geographically remote, some are newish, some are very old. The oldest prison is in Invercargill, which opened in 1910.

The World Prison Brief for June 2020 shows the New Zealand prison rate is at 188 per 100,000 head of population, which is the lowest it has been for some time. It's not as high as the USA, at 639 per 100,000, but it's higher than our Aussie neighbours at 111, or Canada at 107, or the UK at 118. If this data is disaggregated, the ethnic disparities are stark. The Māori incarceration rate was 685 per 100,000 at the end of 2019. At the time of writing (in 2020), 52 per cent of New Zealand prisoners were Māori, 30 per cent European, 12 per cent Pasifika, 5 per cent Asian.

This data shows significant ethnic disparities in imprisonment, leading many to conclude that our justice system is not as colour-blind as might be expected. When such disproportionate figures exist, it is hard to explain this as simply 'do the crime, do the time'. The endnotes deliver hard facts that are stark and sobering.[14] There is recognition that our current justice system, created by Europeans using a European blueprint, and with an individualistic, punitive mindset, is just not working for Māori New Zealanders.

The Department of Corrections embarked on the Hōkai Rangi strategy in 2019, a five-year plan that seeks to turn around the imbalanced incarceration statistics for Māori. At its heart, this strategy seeks to uphold a Māori proverb: 'Kotahi anō te kaupapa: ko te oranga o te iwi; There is only one purpose to our work: the wellness and well-being of people.' Increased emphasis is being placed on partnership; on providing a service that is humanising and healing rather than punitive; on incorporating a te ao Māori world view; on involving whānau where possible; and on looking at whakapapa to give a sense of prideful identity rather than a clouding sense of shame. Know who you are so you know where you are going. The cogs turn slowly, especially in government organisations, but initiatives such as these, increasingly spearheaded by Māori, are a step in the right direction.

The current picture in our prisons nonetheless remains bleak. Poverty, childhood toxic stress, drug use and gang membership sluice people towards incarceration. Socio-medical factors, which have a large degree of overlap and in some cases may be caused by environmental factors, also contribute. Issues include mental illness, domestic and sexual violence, head injuries, and genetic changes caused by toxic stress.

In 2020, almost 38 per cent of prisoners had gang connections; the police recorded more than 7000 patched or prospective gang members in the country. This is an increase of 50 per cent in just three years. It appears that New Zealand gangs are recruiting members faster than the police.

Gangs have existed here for decades. Pacific Islanders banded together as the King Cobras in the 1950s; Pākehā formed skinhead gangs in the 1970s; Māori formed the Mongrel Mob, Black Power and the Nomads that same decade. Gang membership increased in the 1970s due to recession, but after the 1980s numbers dropped and gang activity became low-key. A government-funded group employment scheme was hugely successful in reducing numbers. Then, in 2011, the Rebel motorcycle gang arrived on these shores. They ran a slick recruitment campaign, emphasising bling – Rolls Royces, flash motorbikes. This sophisticated look attracted new members in droves, and other gangs scrambled to keep up. Gang members such as Jade and Matt are often the products of difficult backgrounds, looking for belonging and friendship. Yet gangs also cause significant misery and fallout, leaving victims, addicts and violence in their wake.

Trade in methamphetamine has skyrocketed. A survey conducted in 2017 indicated that 3.1 per cent of respondents had used it; by extrapolation, 138,000 New Zealanders. A staggering 1.8 tonnes of meth was seized by police and customs in 2019 – thrice as much as in 2018. Meth has many street names: speed, crack, P, ice, crank, go, pure, chalk. It is increasingly used by professionals, builders and tradespeople, and can lead to addiction after just one use in some people. It releases a massive amount of dopamine, which causes feelings of pleasure and improves motivation, memory retention and learning. Ongoing usage can lead to sore-riddled greyish skin, structural damage to the heart, stroke, loss of muscle mass from malnutrition, and poor muscular coordination. Withdrawal leads to insomnia, anger, irritability and the craving for more meth.

A 2015 Department of Corrections study of 1200 prisoners found high rates of mental ill-health that were often undetected, under-reported and under-treated. This was the first time in 17 years that such a study had been conducted. It is a stark reminder that patients who are prisoners have much more complexity to their presentation than the general population.[15] For example, the study found that 91 per cent of prisoners surveyed had a lifetime diagnosis of a mental-health disorder. Rates for anxiety, depression, post-traumatic stress disorder and substance abuse were all significantly higher than they were for non-prisoners. Rates of mental-health issues were worse for female than male prisoners.

Traumatic brain injuries (TBIs) are a significant source of ongoing dysfunction in sufferers. The human brain is capable of much creativity and output, given the right circumstances. There's so much potential cocooned inside and so many ways that potential can be suffocated. Damage to the brain can have life-long sequelae. Many studies have found that TBIs are common among prisoners (possibly almost two-thirds of male prisoners may be thus afflicted), with the vast majority unrecognised.[16] Some, especially those who experience multiple injuries over time, can develop post-concussion syndrome. Most sufferers of TBI recover after one year; there is evidence that some people with repeated TBI may have ongoing symptoms for years.

The front and sides of the brain are particularly sensitive to injury. This can result in quite specific impairments, such as: poor hearing, language difficulties leading to poor comprehension and expression, delayed understanding of and reaction to information, moodiness or irritability, impulsiveness or aggression, disorganised thoughts and behaviour so that the sufferer seems 'all over the place', and apathy. Having a head injury doubles the likelihood of a mental-health issue, and TBI sufferers are found to have higher rates of substance abuse. The links between TBI, mental illness and criminality are complex. More research is needed to establish clear causal pathways. Additionally, while there are no comprehensive studies in New Zealand that look at the incidence of developmental disorders such as dyslexia or autism in prisoners, it is useful to look at figures from overseas; see endnote.[17]

The Department of Corrections estimates that 60 per cent of prisoners have literacy and numeracy skills below that of Level 1 competency in the National Certificate in Educational Achievement (NCEA). Sixty-six per cent have no formal qualifications, which impacts future employment potential and retraining.

Lastly, as discussed more extensively in Dr Jin Russell's chapter, there is much evidence that toxic stress in childhood, such as that due to chronic poverty or family violence, can lead to structural changes in our brains. Children exposed to toxic stress grow up with brains that are preprogrammed to be on high alert for threats, to seek pleasurable activities that numb pain, and to make poor decisions because of an underdeveloped decision-making centre. The expression of their genetic code can be altered, perpetuating these issues for generations. All of these factors point to a complex interplay of health as well as criminogenic issues in those who are incarcerated.

In the 1970s and 1980s, there was a 'nothing works' mentality when it came to rehabilitating prisoners. Nowadays, plenty of national and international evidence indicates that psychological treatment programmes can be very effective. However, due to funding and time constraints, not enough prisoners will have access to psychotherapy, especially those on remand or on short sentences. Many of the treatment programmes have a cognitive behavioural therapy (CBT) focus. There are certain programmes that seem to have quite good outcomes, such as those with sexual offenders. CBT can reduce rates of reoffending by up to 40 per cent, and the frequency and seriousness of offences of those who are reconvicted are also reduced. Currently, the use of CBT for youth offenders is only 10 per cent that of adult offenders, but there is strong international evidence that expanding this would help reduce crime.

***

Catarina's work can be arduous. The interview rooms in the prison are small, they lack privacy, and they are not particularly welcoming. There are no couches or soft furnishings, no inspirational quotes on the walls or personal family photos of the therapist to provide a sense of intimacy or vulnerability. There are just windows in internal doors, and cameras so that security can intervene if things get out of hand. Nonetheless, there is a long list of prisoners waiting to see Catarina. Trauma therapists who work in prison are a rare breed, yet the incidence of significant trauma among prisoners is disproportionately high.

'Eighty per cent or more of those whom I see have undiagnosed PTSD. There is inevitably a history of physical or sexual abuse. Or else the flipside of abuse – neglect. Children who do not receive adequate emotional nourishment do not grow up to become healthy adults. Usually, by adulthood, self-esteem is non-existent. Hopelessness is a big issue.'

Catarina takes an unconventional 'intelligent love' approach. She decided early on in her career that the traditional 'receiving arms' image of counselling did not seem to work well with many clients. 'The quote I use often and which people love is: "If you always do what you've always done, you will always get what you've always got." It really gets people thinking.

'Right from the start, I adapt firm rules and set clear boundaries. I instigate time out when necessary. I advise my clients that I am highly experienced. They like hearing that – it gives them security, helps to build trust. I tell them that I have strong bones: I will put firm rules around the therapeutic relationship and I will talk tough with them when I need to. But I also have soft flesh: I will hear their pain and I will try to help.'

Catarina gives the client a chance to learn a little bit about her. 'I say to them, if you're interested in why I became a trauma therapist, it is because I have suffered trauma myself. If they seem interested, I tell them a bit more. I say, I healed and learnt how to live with the memories. There is hope. Things can change. I am an expert in trauma therapy, but *you* are the expert in your own life. How about we work together?'

It takes a long time to get to the core of what matters. Fundamentally, Catarina says, the crime committed against these women has never been addressed, and so Catarina validates, she revisits, she searches for their buried dignity as a human being.

Catarina elucidates that Jade has PTSD, a result of her childhood abuse, fractured social situation and the traumatic death of her partner. It is manifested in flashbacks, nightmares, repetitive distressing images, constant negative thoughts. Her abuse of alcohol and meth are part of the self-destructive behaviour seen in PTSD sufferers. Over several sessions, Catarina pinpoints how the trauma has created distorted thinking, chronic depression and anxiety, and maladaptive behaviour patterns. She helps Jade with thinking and behavioural skills to manage her anxiety and anger, using a combination of psychoeducation, cognitive behavioural therapy, guided retelling of her trauma, validation of her story and her worth, and lots of reassurance. She also focuses on Jade's addictions, and provides her with practical tools for dealing with these, for example, referral to onsite programmes such as Kowhiritanga.

Being in prison with access to trauma therapy gives Jade the opportunity to treat her anxiety and her PTSD, to understand her addictions, and to think about a new way forward. The words of the American lawyer and social justice activist Bryan Stevenson are poignant when applied to Jade and other prisoners: 'Each of us is more than the worst thing we've ever done.'

A grumpy man

patient: Willie*; nurse: Ria*

There is a Māori man called Willie in Room 5, but the nursing staff in the cardiothoracic surgical ward are avoiding him. Willie is in his seventies. He's in a foul mood. He's been swearing at the nurses. At times he is verbose, spouting a tirade of abuse; at other times, he's sullen and recalcitrant. The nurses are having a hard time getting him to take his medications. All those life-saving tablets that will squeeze and sculpt his weakened heart back into shape, if only he'd swallow them.

Nurse Ria* is working an extra shift today as a bureau, or temporary cover, nurse. Sometimes bureau nurses get 'dumped with the grumps' – tasked with looking after the difficult patients. Ria is asked to look after Willie.

'Kia ora, Willie. My name's Ria. I'll be your nurse today,' she says as she walks up to the patient's bed.

'Kia ora,' he says. He flicks a look her way, then returns to staring at the TV screen. His face is set in a staunch 'I'm-not-interested' vibe. Ria can tell that he's not really watching the TV.

There are three other patients sharing this four-bed room in Greenlane Hospital. The smell of disinfectant rises from the newly cleaned linoleum floors. Soon goose-necked bottles full of urine will need to be emptied, bedpans cleaned out. Then it will be time for the morning nursing rounds: checking observations on each patient and dispensing medications.

'You probably think I'm Māori, eh, koro? But I'm not. I'm a Cook Islander.' Ria smooths the bedcovers, checks Willie's pulse and blood pressure and keeps up a light banter as she works. She hopes that by calling him koro, an affectionate Māori term for an older male relative, it will help her make some sort of a connection with Willie.

'Oh, okay then.' Willie continues to stare at the TV. His face is lined and he looks tired. He is not a big man. In fact, he looks frail and defenceless. His skinny legs stretch out under the covers, his smallish paunch rises and falls as he breathes.

'Where are you from, Willie?' Ria asks.

'Gisborne.'

'Oh yeah? That's a long way, huh?'

'Yep. Been here two bloody weeks.' Willie scowls at her.

Ria had read Willie's notes earlier during handover. He'd collapsed at the supermarket and was rushed to Gisborne

Hospital, where he was assessed with blood tests, an electrocardiogram (a recording of the electrical activity of the heart) and an echocardiogram (an ultrasound of the heart to evaluate structure and blood flow), all of which confirmed a significant heart attack.

A heart attack occurs from the build-up of fatty deposits inside the arteries that supply blood to the heart. There are umpteen factors that influence this: poor physical activity, smoking, obesity, diabetes, genetics, ethnicity, gender. The internal lining of the coronary artery is damaged by the build-up of these deposits, and smooth muscle cells move in to help patch the damage. This attracts cholesterol, other fats and white blood cells. Eventually a plaque develops. Over time this plaque becomes calcified and scarred, in the process of atherosclerosis. Because the artery is narrowed, less blood flows to the heart muscle, causing chest pain (angina). Sometimes these plaque-like deposits rupture and create an occluding blood clot. Blood flow to a part of the heart then drops steeply, leading to a myocardial infarction, or death of heart tissue. The sudden blockage can also cause an irregular heart rhythm, which increases the likelihood of death.

Willie was airlifted to Greenlane Hospital for further treatment because, in the early 2000s when Willie had this heart attack, Gisborne Hospital did not have the facilities to provide the cardiac care needed. He underwent a coronary angiogram via an incision in his groin, and a thin, flexible catheter was threaded in through his femoral artery, through his abdominal aorta, to his heart. The tip of the catheter was placed in his left main-stem coronary artery initially, then his right coronary artery. Each time dye spurted out of the tip, X-rays were taken. These showed significant blockages in all three of his arteries.

Willie needed a coronary artery bypass graft (CABG). The long saphenous vein was harvested from his inner left leg. Then a central cut on his chest wall, down through his sternum, allowed the two halves of his ribcage to be cracked open to enable access to his heart. After his heart was stopped with medication, a heart–lung bypass machine oxygenated his blood and pumped it around his body. The cardiac surgeons cut out the diseased heart arteries, stitched sections of leg vein into place, then sewed the breastbone back with wire, and restarted Willie's heart. He was moved to the cardiovascular intensive care unit, and once he was more stable, he was put in the cardiothoracic surgical ward where Ria met him.

***

In the past, prior to the existence of good medical and surgical treatments for heart disease, there was an uptick of deaths from cardiovascular disease. This was particularly true between the 1950s and 1970s, coinciding with changed diets, reduced levels of activity and increased rates of smoking. Conversely, heart disease was a rare phenomenon at the start of the twentieth century.

The advent of CABGs and other interventions saw deaths from cardiovascular disease fall in the 1980s and 1990s. Currently, cardiovascular disease (heart attacks, strokes and blood vessel disease) are still the leading cause of death in New Zealanders – almost one in three deaths. The rates for cardiovascular disease are even worse for Māori – twice the death rate compared to non-Māori, with one and a half times the hospitalisation rates. Cardiovascular disease is the leading cause of death for Pasifika peoples.

Recovery from CABG surgery will often take several weeks, and up to three months. It flattens patients physically and mentally. To improve his heart health, Willie's been started on several medications: a statin to lower his cholesterol; aspirin to reduce the chance of blood clots causing further occlusions; a beta blocker, now that he is stable, to improve the long-term contractility of his heart. These tablets are important to give Willie's damaged heart the best chance of recovery. However, he has been disinterested in his healthcare, downright hostile at times. Low mood is common after heart surgery, as is extreme fatigue and pain from wound sites. The other staff have largely assumed that this is what is causing Willie's obstreperousness.

. Ria checks Willie's wounds. His sternal scar drops like a zipper line from his collarbone to the lower end of his breastbone. His left leg also has a scar from his groin down to his ankle, the site of the saphenous vein harvest. Both wounds look healthy.

'So who lives at home with you, Willie?' Ria keeps chatting as she works around him. As a Pasifika New Zealander, she is cognisant of the importance of family in people's lives.

Willie's face slackens. He looks down at the sheets. He is trying not to cry. 'My boy. My moko, Tawhiri*. I'm his koro. He's only five, you know. I've looked after him since he was born. I've been here for weeks. I haven't been able to check on him.'

The patient's defences dissolve. Ria sees that Willie is tense and worried about his grandson. This realisation comes with a sense of frustration that he has been in hospital for days, yet no one appears to have asked him for the one thing he most wants to do.

'Aw, Willie, that's so hard not knowing if he's okay, eh?' Ria says.

'Yep.'

'Shall I try and see if we can get hold of Tawhiri for you?'

'Oh, please!'

Ria finishes her nursing rounds. She liaises with the charge nurse, then arranges a collect call to one of Willie's relatives in Gisborne. Someone tracks down the little boy. As Willie chats to his mokopuna, his face lights up. He smiles, he nods, he laughs. He is a changed man. The phone call lasts just 20 minutes, but it is perhaps the most healing 20 minutes Willie has experienced since his heart attack.

***

Ria's parents arrived in New Zealand from the Cook Islands some decades ago. They brought with them a determination to work hard and to forge a new life for their nascent family.

They found work making asbestos cladding, yet neither they nor their fellow workers were aware that research in the 1930s had already found cases of asbestosis in workers exposed to it, with subsequent clear links to the development of mesothelioma (a malignant tumour that can form in the lining of the lungs, abdomen or heart). To Ria's parents, it was simply a steady job.

The infamous Dawn Raids – police raids on the homes and workplaces of suspected overstayers – began in 1976 and continued until the 1980s. Although Pacific Islanders made up only one-third of overstayers (the majority were from Great Britain, Australia and South Africa), they made up almost 90 per cent of those arrested. During this time, when Ria's father caught the bus to work, he hid behind a raised newspaper. He couldn't read English, but he wanted to avoid eye contact with white people so as not to cause offence or draw attention.

The family bought their first home after a few years of saving: a rambling weatherboard house, with enough land to grow taro and bananas. They were the second Pasifika family in the street. The house was never locked. It was a safe childhood growing up there – an abundance of rain and sun, the cloying smell of gardenia, a dearth of traffic.

When Ria was 14, a relative suffered a seizure in front of her. 'I desperately wanted to be able to help him,' she says, 'but I couldn't. I was immobilised by fear. I resolved never to be in that position again.' It was Ria's first catalyst towards a career in nursing. The second catalyst was her father's ill health with diabetes, and later lung cancer. The photos of him when he was younger showed a fit young Cook Islander who worked the soil of his island home and lived off fresh produce. He was not a smoker, but it is likely that his changed diet and lifestyle in New Zealand helped trigger his diabetes. His workplace exposure to asbestos probably led to his lung cancer.

Ria intuitively knew, during her training and later while working as a newly minted nurse, that it was essential to incorporate a patient's culture into their care. Willie's story became a perfect example of the importance of maintaining a culturally centred model of care. This allows for holistic care that is patient-centred and empowering, especially at a time when a patient is vulnerable and relying on other people to get them through.

'My colleagues and nursing students have tears in their eyes when I retell Willie's story. It reminds them of their own grandparents. That emotional connection is the trigger that leads to the action of remembering to treat their patients holistically, as if every patient is their own grandparent. It's important for medical staff to recognise the impact of mental, relational and spiritual health on physical health. This is fundamental to the Pasifika model of health.

'Patients don't always realise how much they affect staff. We think we are the ones doing all the giving, handing out meds, looking after physical needs and so on. But patients frequently give back intangible but priceless things in return. It wasn't until years later that I recognised the reciprocity of Willie's story, how he'd given me this golden example of looking after the whole person, not just the disease. Willie's story has become part of my narrative. He's passed on now, but I still refer to him as my dear koro.'

***

Health practitioners who have a good understanding of and appreciation for culture can bring a profound richness to patient interactions. It helps make health encounters less transactional and more relational, more healing. Good health encounters are particularly important for ethnicities that do not have equitable health outcomes in New Zealand.

Pasifika New Zealanders make up the fourth-largest ethnic group in New Zealand, behind European, Māori and Asian ethnic groups. In the latest 2018 census, they make up 8 per cent of the population, or roughly 350,000 people. More than half are born here, and have made the transition from new immigrants to third-generation New Zealanders. Most Pasifika New Zealanders are also young, with a median age of 22, and are more likely to be multilingual than other New Zealanders.

They are a diverse group. Forty ethnicities, eight main ones: Samoan, Cook Islands Māori, Tongan, Niuean, Fijian, Tokelauan, Tuvaluan and I-Kiribati. About two-thirds of Pasifika New Zealanders reside in Auckland. While their birth rate is dropping, it remains higher than the New Zealand average. This group of New Zealanders is making great strides in representation in all sorts of areas. Pasifika New Zealanders are more likely than other Kiwis to volunteer their time to help others. They are more likely to vote if they are eligible. They bring a colourful diversity to New Zealand society.

However, significant issues remain, many of which then impinge on health outcomes.[18] Lower incomes, higher rates of unemployment, poorer and more crowded housing, fewer assets, higher rates of chronic illness – that desperate, familiar litany. In high-density, poorer suburbs, some people resort to living in cold garages, with thin roofs that thunder in rainstorms. Mould casts lace-like patterns on walls and ceilings. Multigenerational families crowd into small homes. Often older relatives are not sent to a nursing home as per cultural expectations; this takes up time and resources for cash-strapped families. Crowding has a knock-on effect on education. The rates of Pasifika in tertiary education or with a qualification of some sort remains significantly lower than for other ethnic groups, although, in recent years, these gaps are narrowing.

Even more disturbing are the lower rates of referral from health practitioners for much-needed higher-level care. It's an inequity that is invisible until analysis makes it clear, and issues persist despite Pasifika people turning up to GP appointments at higher rates than others. There is a veritable epidemic of diabetes, obesity and metabolic syndrome hitting Pacific Islanders, not just in Western countries such as New Zealand but also in the islands themselves. This epidemic afflicts Indigenous groups around the world. We see the same story in Māori, in Australian

Aborigines and Torres Strait Islanders, in First Nations people in the Americas and in the Indigenous groups of Asia.

It might be easy to ascribe these medical issues to poor lifestyle choices. There is some element of choice involved. There are also environmental, genetic and epigenetic triggers at work. As Dr Caldwell Esselstyn, an American physician and former Olympic rowing champion, says: 'Genetics loads the gun, lifestyle pulls the trigger.' Various studies have ascertained that genetic causes may be responsible for 40–70 per cent of obesity. Often, multiple genes predisposing to obesity (including the fat mass and obesity-associated gene FTO) can be found in overweight people. These can work in tandem to increase hunger levels and caloric intake, reduce satiety, reduce activity levels and increase the tendency to store fat. It's a complex interplay, though. Genetics alone won't automatically lead to obesity. Rather, the environment, food choices and activity levels modulate the expression of these genes. There is likely also an epigenetic component whereby certain genes in our bodies are switched on or off depending on our environment. Stressful environments can lead to maladaptive genes being turned on. Some studies have shown that certain Pasifika populations may have alterations in the leptin gene, which regulates satiety.

Pacific Islanders genetically have more uric acid in their systems (this is seen in pre-European-contact skeletal remains, which sometimes show gouty lesions). A preponderance of uric acid causes gout and predisposes to metabolic syndrome – a cluster of conditions that occur together, including increased blood pressure, high blood sugar, excess body fat around the waist and around the liver, and abnormal cholesterol or triglyceride levels. There's evidence that uric acid can alter the function of cellular mitochondria, tiny organelles that help regulate energy production in our bodies. Put simply, high uric-acid levels can increase our susceptibility to obesity.

Some theories propose that contact with European cultures, and the resulting loss of life on some Pacific islands due to Western infectious diseases such as measles (up to 75 per cent of the population of some islands) may have reduced genetic diversity among Pasifika populations. The survivors may have been those more predisposed to metabolic syndrome, diabetes and obesity.

As mentioned in patient Arama's story, the World Health Organization has recognised colonisation, or even just contact with Europeans, as the most significant social determinant of health affecting Indigenous peoples worldwide. Consider these historical atrocities, the reverberations of which are still felt today: the outlawing of Indigenous gatherings; the forced relocations of communities; forbidding Indigenous languages from being spoken; discriminatory child-welfare legislation. Many of these practices severed the connection of people to their land, and led to intergenerational mental-health and familial effects.

Changed diet is another significant culprit. Certain foods, and in particular fructose found in high-fructose corn syrup, are a major driver of the metabolic processes that lead to fat storage. Wealthier nations are culpable in this regard. Not only do soft-drink companies export their products to the islands, they also have factories there due to the low cost of labour. New Zealand and the US export cheap fatty meat such as lamb flaps, lard and turkey tails to the islands because there is limited domestic demand for these items. This has been described as the export of non-communicable diseases from wealthier nations to the Pacific. The bottom line is profit, not peoples' lives.

Disparities in health persist even when factors such as poverty, education and location are eliminated. This highlights the importance of culturally centred healthcare, so that health practitioners can fully understand their patients and walk alongside them, rather than talking at cross-purposes to them.

Ria found that the most significant thing impeding Willie's progress was his anguish at being cut off from his grandson, and the difference in his subsequent progress once this was recognised was astounding. He started gunning it to get home. And in the same way that some patients feel more comfortable with a female versus a male health practitioner, finding a medic who you can relate to on a cultural level is important. Presently only about 2 per cent of doctors in New Zealand are of Pasifika ethnicity.

Pasifika peoples see health and wellness as a gift, incorporating physical, mental, social and spiritual well-being. Good health allows them to be more productive members of the community. Being unhealthy brings shame and embarrassment. There are several models of Pasifika health, such as Fonua (Tongan) and Fonofale (Samoan, Cook Islander, Tongan, Niuean, Tokelaun and Fijian). These models are more holistic than the typical approach a Western-trained physician might take, as they acknowledge the overriding importance of family, culture and spirituality to our physical and mental health.

***

Cultural competency is essential for high-quality healthcare. Practitioners who ask about and are aware of their Pasifika patients' health-related beliefs have been shown to offer improved care. Pasifika patients often defer to authority figures, and until they have built a close rapport with their doctor or nurse, they are highly unlikely to question advice or treatment, or reveal their true health status. It takes time and patience to get past that 'Yes, doctor' reply that divulges so little.

Family and community are much more important than they are in more individualistic Western societies. Relationships with the wider community and professionals are characterised by generosity and integrity. Huge importance is placed on behaviour that is good for the community, not just for the individual. Often the role of the patient is to passively accept medical treatment, while their family members advocate on their behalf. This familial advocacy is important to acknowledge and incorporate into the healthcare package, as it can lead to more effective health interventions for the patient. For Pasifika people, 'the way things are done' is important, for example, fa'a Samoa (the Samoan way) dictates how Samoans should behave with regard to their family, community and church. Respect is important, especially towards those of higher social status, such as ministers, doctors and politicians.

The importance of holistic care was cruelly brought home to Ria when her older brother got sick. A chest X-ray in 2017 picked up a shadow on his lungs – a significant finding in a smoker: incipient cancer lurking in the bronchial tree. The hospital could not get hold of him and he was 'lost to follow-up'. Eventually the cancer spread to his brain; he died in 2019. Ria desperately wishes that the hospital staff had tried harder to contact extended family. If they had, they might have learnt that her brother had a wife who was a meth addict, and that he was the sole carer of several children, his time consumed by school runs, cooking meals, doctor's visits. That's why he was hard to get hold of. His whānau, had they known the situation, would have advocated for him, helped him get to his appointments, looked after the kids.

Another case, which came before the Health and Disability Commissioner, involved a quiet, gentle Samoan man who did not drink. He was at a party and tried to break up a fight. He got hit in the head, losing consciousness for several minutes, and was then taken by ambulance to ED. His wife went with him. By this time, he was acting oddly, muttering, lashing out. It was assumed by staff that he was just intoxicated, having been at a party. A blood-alcohol level was not done. It was also assumed he was muttering in Samoan, when in fact his speech was incoherent to his wife. She did not want to make a fuss; he'd already been assessed by the doctor. The man subsequently died of a bleed in the brain – something that could have been prevented with attention and perceptivity instead of assumptions.

Many of the health issues facing Pasifika peoples are preventable with relatively easy interventions – better insulation for homes, better nutrition for children, restrictions on harmful foods – all of which would have significant positive impacts for the whole of society. Ria and other health practitioners are increasingly recognising the vital importance of culturally centred care that treats all patients as if they are part of the practitioner's own family – with compassion, respect and recognition of the wider context in which they live.

PART 3

Time proves everything

A fat bomb a day keeps the doctor away

patient: Sarona Rameka; neurologist: Dr Matthew Phillips

At the age of 37, Sarona is expecting her first child. The loveliness of expectation is overwhelming. It's 2017, and Sarona and her husband, Vern, have just bought a new home, near the waters of Lake Taupō. Two teenagers are also living in the house – Vern's son from a previous relationship, and a niece, both of whom are excited about the impending arrival. They don't even try to appear nonchalant, but fall over themselves to help.

Sarona and her husband feel unprepared and disorganised. 'I thought I had a few weeks up my sleeve because it was a planned induction,' says Sarona, 'so I was still working as a marketing consultant. I was going to get newborn clothes soon. We had a bassinet, a car seat, a rocker. I had an Ed Hardy bag for all the baby stuff, and some cowhide slippers.'

Sarona, who is part Samoan and part English, has had myasthenia gravis (MG) for more than a decade. Back when she was 26, when she was training for the New Zealand kickboxing team, she noted that her muscles felt terribly weak after training. She thought she must have been just overdoing it and that some rest would fix her. However, her symptoms got worse. Her facial muscles started to droop. She was initially misdiagnosed as having Bell's palsy, but after further tests was diagnosed with MG. She was treated with pyridostigmine, prednisone and intermittent courses of intravenous immunoglobulin (IVIg), and was eventually put on long-term azathioprine.

She was also found at the time to have a mediastinal mass in her chest (the mediastinum is the anatomical region sandwiched between the lungs, and contains the heart, thymus gland, trachea, oesophagus and other structures). The mass was surgically removed in 2007, via laparoscopic (keyhole) surgery. Histology revealed a type B2 invasive thymoma. Every time Sarona had a relapse of her MG, she needed almost three months of IVIg infusions to help her improve.

MG is a chronic autoimmune, neuromuscular condition affecting voluntary muscles (but not involuntary muscles such as those in the heart and digestive tract). It affects perhaps 14 out of 100,000 people in New Zealand, and life expectancy is normal. The usual symptoms of this disorder are unexplained muscle weakness that increases during periods of activity and improves after rest. It often impacts the muscles that control eye and lid movement, the facial muscles for expression, and those involved in chewing, talking and swallowing. Sometimes MG affects the muscles of the limbs, those in the neck, and the muscles that help us to breathe.

In normal muscle function, when an electrical impulse travels down a motor nerve, the nerve endings release a neurotransmitter called acetylcholine. This then binds to receptors on the muscle, which kickstart the contraction of the muscle cell. In MG, this process is awry. The body's immune system mistakenly attacks its own cells: naturally produced antibodies block, alter or destroy the acetylcholine receptors, preventing the muscle from working.

The thymus gland, which sits behind the upper end of the breastbone like a squishy pendant, is involved in training immune cells to behave properly. It normally shrinks during puberty, however, in many people with MG, the thymus gland remains enlarged. In 10 to 30 per cent of patients with MG, a thymoma will develop, as it did in Sarona. A thymoma is composed largely of benign (non-cancerous) cells but it can, albeit rarely, become malignant.

Treatment of MG is varied. Cholinesterase inhibitors such as pyridostigmine can help stop the normal breakdown of acetylcholine. Immunosuppressive drugs such as azathioprine can help block the formation of abnormal antibodies – Sarona was treated with this for almost a decade. Plasmapheresis can sieve out abnormal antibodies from the blood. High dose IVIg suppresses the immune system's production of abnormal antibodies, while providing the body with normal antibodies from donated blood. Some people get better by themselves. For others, thymectomies (removal of the thymus) can help dramatically.

When Sarona's eyelids start to droop during her pregnancy, she realises she's getting another MG relapse. Then she develops shortness of breath and pleuritic chest pain (pain felt when breathing in), so she checks in with her neurologist, Dr Matthew (Matt) Phillips, in March 2017. She's 32 weeks through her pregnancy. She's been his patient since 2016, and theirs is a perfunctory relationship.

Matt checks Sarona over. 'I'll cover you with a five-day course of IVIg for the myasthenia symptoms, which will last you six to eight weeks,' he says. 'If your shortness of breath worsens, it will be important to get a chest X-ray.' Matt arranges to see Sarona again after she delivers because he won't be involved in her obstetric care.

The mild MG symptoms improve with the IVIg, but the shortness of breath worsens. Sarona feels like there is something sitting on her chest: a sack full of lead, refusing to move. There are sharp, stabbing chest pains every time she breathes in. She turns up to ED twice and twice she is told, 'It's just the baby pushing upwards.' But one week before her planned induction, her midwife, increasingly concerned by Sarona's breathlessness, demands she get a chest X-ray. The films reveal several masses in her left chest. The largest is 10×5×14 centimetres. Collectively, the masses are the size of a football. They were not present on Sarona's last X-ray, three years before, and are a sinister, alien presence. A CT scan reveals a large tumour with extensive spread – it abuts her pericardium (the sac-like covering around the heart), and is invading the left pleura (the membrane covering the lung).

An urgent caesarean section is organised. Sarona's newborn ends up in the neonatal intensive care unit due to some minor breathing issues. A guided biopsy of Sarona's mass confirms a thymoma, type AB, stage IVA (this means that the tumour consists of a combination of cancer cells and white blood cells mixed together, and that it is an advanced cancer that has spread beyond the thymus to other tissue).

The oncology team visit Sarona. The news is not good. As she nurtures her new baby girl, Sarona must face the reality that her own life may only last another six to twelve months – best-case scenario. There is no cure for stage IV thymoma. The only feasible treatment option is palliative chemotherapy to manage tumour-related symptoms. This might buy her those six months but with attendant, debilitating side effects. Radiotherapy is not an option. The oncologists recommend that chemo needs to start within two weeks, however, the first appointment available on the public system is one month away.

When Sarona and Vern pay for a private oncology appointment to get a second opinion, to see if they can fast-track treatment, the news is the same: palliative treatment only, no hope of a cure. They are advised to await the public oncology appointment.

The couple feel that their backs are against the wall. The situation is bleak, horrific, unreal. Just a few weeks ago, they were planning the arrival of their first child together and juggling parental leave, now they are having to contemplate the unthinkable. Sarona and Vern have a strong Christian faith, so they pray hard and ask God to open doors for them. They also start looking into alternative treatments, which is not something they've ever done before but they are desperate. 'The thought of palliative chemotherapy that would leave me terribly fatigued with lots of side effects while not actually curing me did not appeal at all. What was the point? I needed to look after two teenagers and a new baby. I didn't want this to be their last memories of me.'

Sarona starts on an alkaline diet for two weeks, eating according to a dietary plan on the internet that advocates 'alkaline' foods in order to counteract bodily 'acidity', but the information is contradictory, frustrating. Two days prior to the oncology appointment, Sarona's appointment with Dr Phillips rolls around, and she almost cancels. The MG is the least of her worries.

'When I told Matt about my diagnosis, he was visibly shocked. I have never seen a medical professional have so much concern and empathy at a patient's bad news.' Sarona tells him that palliative chemo is her only option, but that she's not particularly keen to go ahead with it.

Matt asks, 'So what will you do?'

'We've researched different therapies. Right now I'm on an alkaline diet,' Sarona tells him. She shrugs and sighs. 'I've read up on some stuff ... I have no idea if it will work, but we have to fight. I'll be seeing the oncologist in two days' time. I'll check in with him also.'

Matt tells Sarona that he's been interested in the effects of ketogenic diets and fasting for several years now and practises the regimens himself. He's done some reading on the metabolic nature of cancer, how it's essentially the body's own cells going AWOL and how there is a theory that depriving cancer cells of energy can kill them. There's plenty of trials where short-term metabolic therapies have been used alongside traditional chemotherapy, to good effect. 'But, look, I don't want to tread on toes,' he says. 'Talk to your oncologist, make your own mind up. If you do decide to trial a metabolic approach to this, I'd be happy to help.'

Sarona remembers how blunt the oncologist was: 'He said that I had zero chance of beating this thing. In hindsight, I'm glad he was so stark. If he'd offered even the smallest glimmer of hope, I would've grabbed it, tried the chemo. As it was, I felt like I literally had nothing to lose, so I told him that I was going to decline the chemo, and try fasting and a ketogenic diet instead. He was extremely sceptical, but he realised that it was a choice I wanted to make. I felt like my life depended on it. Which it did, really.'

So, just five weeks after giving birth, Sarona starts a ten-day fast on the advice of Matt and his own nutrition specialist, Deborah Murtagh. Sarona takes water and salts and some bone broth, but nothing else. She feels terrible by day two. Shivery, grumpy, in pain all over her body, cold. She's snappish and irritable. She drinks plenty of fluids to keep hydrated. She temporarily reduces activity in order to conserve what energy she has.

Fasting can help kickstart our immune system. Unfortunately, this also means that Sarona's dysfunctional MG antibodies are spurred into action. She has a relapse of her MG and is admitted to hospital on day seven of the fast for yet another course of IVIg. To counteract any glucose from the IVIg, her fast is extended to 12 days.

'It was all or nothing at this point. It was scary how fast the myasthenia relapsed, but this was my only therapy to fight the tumour so I wanted to give it everything.'

After finishing the water-only fast, Sarona then switches to a modified ketogenic diet, made up of 60 per cent fat, 30 per cent protein, 5 per cent fibre and just 5 per cent carbohydrate. She eats lots of green vegetables, some meat, eggs, nuts, seeds, creams and natural oils; raw fish with coconut cream; quiches lined with spinach; pizza bases made with almond flour; and 'fat bombs' made up of coconut oil or unsweetened cocoa to help elevate her fat intake. She decides to do a seven-day fast every two months, and eats a modified ketogenic diet in between the fasts. Dr Phillips is there to give her advice and encouragement.

The oncologist arranges a CT scan at the four-month mark. There is no change in tumour size. Sarona has significant diarrhoea, thought to be an autoimmune side effect of the thymoma. She also develops another MG relapse. She's put on IVIg for four months. The eight-month CT scan reveals a 32 per cent reduction in the tumour mass and it is thought the

IVIg may have contributed to this shrinkage as well. However, the next scan at the 12-month mark shows that the tumour has increased again to what it was at diagnosis. Importantly, though, it is now one year post-diagnosis and Sarona is still alive, without having had any chemotherapy.

Sarona increases the frequency of seven-day fasting to once every month instead of once every two months. Each time, she loses about 4 kilos, then regains this when she starts eating again, but now Sarona finds that the side effects of fasting (the muscle pains, the fatigue) do not recur and neither are there side effects from the maintenance ketogenic diet.

But at 25 months, in July 2019, a CT scan shows that the tumour has increased in size by 13 per cent. Things take a significant downturn. Sarona gets uncontrolled diarrhoea for months, she starts losing weight, she gets a severe relapse of her MG, with all four limbs involved, and dysarthria (unclear speech due to weak speech muscles). Overall, she loses 30 per cent of her body weight. Further doses of IVIg do not seem to help. She is admitted to Rotorua, then Waikato Hospital. She goes into respiratory failure because the MG affects her breathing muscles; she is intubated and transferred to intensive care. She stays there for three weeks, getting treated with plasma exchange and more IVIg. The ICU staff try to extubate her twice. Twice they fail. They get ready to extubate her for the third time. They tell Sarona's husband that if this attempt does not work, she will be NFR. Not for resuscitation. The ICU staff reason that someone with an incurable malignancy, who has failed extubation twice, is of poor likelihood of improving.

Sarona's husband rings Matt in a panic. Matt heads straight to ICU. He points out to the ICU medics that, normally, a 38-year-old patient with myasthenia gravis would not be NFR. And although Sarona has a stage IV thymic carcinoma, she has lived for 25 months after her diagnosis. Sarona has, by this stage, also had steroids for several days (not trialled initially because of a previous bad reaction). The third time around, the extubation is successful.

Two months after leaving ICU, Sarona hears some rasping noises in her chest. She gets a chest X-ray done. The radiologist report mentions that the tumour is now 'insignificant'; it has in fact shrunk by 96 per cent. A subsequent CT scan confirms this. Sarona's oncologist, who throughout her trial with fasting and ketogenic diets remained a sceptic, emails her the latest image. The tumour is almost completely gone. He cannot believe it.

Twenty years ago, Sarona had a verse of scripture prayed over her, Jeremiah 29:11. 'For I know the plans I have for you,' declares the Lord, 'Plans to prosper you and not to harm you, plans to give you hope and a future.' Over the course of her battle with the thymoma, Sarona holds on to these words. She is reminded of them, unexpectedly and without prompting, by various people – an aunty, a friend from Christchurch, an uncle. She's watching an episode of *Criminal Minds*, and Spencer Reid quotes the verse. However, she keeps wondering what the plans for her future could possibly look like with a stage IV incurable cancer. How can she prosper? The one thing she holds on to is hope.

Now, four years after her diagnosis, Sarona is leading a full and active life. Her only remaining medication is decreasing doses of prednisone. She knows fasting and a ketogenic diet will be an integral part of her lifestyle for the foreseeable future.

***

Matthew Phillips grew up in British Columbia, Canada. The wilderness of Alaska was an icy hop from his hometown of Terrace; the Pacific coastline was on the western border, a wild, thundering beast, jagged with heavily forested fjords. When he was 26, Matt travelled to Australia and studied medicine at Flinders University in Adelaide, underwent his basic physician training at the Queen Elizabeth in Adelaide, and then spent a further two years in neurology, subspecialising in neurophysiology, at the Royal Melbourne Hospital.

Matt loved neurology – still does – but the avenues of work open to him specialised in a disease or specialised in a diagnostic technique. Both felt too circumscribed. He wanted to focus on treatment, on something curative, on something that would make a difference. Unable to settle, he bought a one-way ticket to Buenos Aires. Amid cries of 'What are ya doing, mate? You're a good neurologist; stop pissing around' from colleagues, he gave away his laptop and phone and took off. He travelled around South America for a year. He rode an old horse called

Miguel in Argentina, was drenched by the Iguaçu Falls, climbed mountains, ran his tongue along the edges of salt flats, and visited stone tables where animal and human sacrifices had occurred.

Back in Australia, he worked in Cairns as a general neurologist. By now increasingly aware of the evidence that fasting and ketogenic diets could reverse Type II diabetes, he took off again, this time to Asia. In a blog, he wrote, 'I'm a free man at the start of a long journey whose conclusion is uncertain.' Somewhere in his meanderings through Sri Lanka, Nepal and Myanmar, a friend told him about a book, *Cancer as a Metabolic Disease: On the origin, management, and prevention of cancer* by Thomas Seyfried, a biochemical geneticist and professor of biology. It expanded on an earlier theory by Otto Warburg (a German medical doctor who won the Nobel Prize in Physiology or Medicine in 1931) that cancer is primarily a metabolic disease, not a genetic one, and hence requires a metabolic approach to treat it. Specifically, the theory goes that all cancers are a disorder in the structure and function of the mitochondria, the organelles inside our cells that help to generate energy. The malfunctioning mitochondria create reactive oxygen species – unstable molecules that can cause damage to DNA, RNA and proteins. Thus, the genetic defects observed in various cancers are a downstream effect of the metabolic abnormalities.

The way to treat cancer, Seyfried argued, is to treat it metabolically. Cancer cells are high users of glucose. Other sources of energy for cancerous cells include glutamine, a type of amino acid, and growth factor, a protein that helps cells to grow and wounds to heal. When we fast, or when we eat ketogenic diets, glucose levels plummet and starve cancer cells of their primary energy source. Glutamine and growth-factor levels also fall. Healthy cells can easily switch to using ketones for their energy needs (ketones are made by our livers out of fat when we are fasting, but they are also made when we are in starvation mode, during prolonged exercise, with alcoholism, or with untreated Type I diabetes). Tumour cells, on the other hand, are unable to utilise ketones. Their altered genes tell these cells to keep multiplying without stopping. This ongoing growth in the face of non-existent energy leads to tumour cell death.

Matt decided to trial fasting and ketogenic diets himself. He did a two-day fast in Myanmar initially, and while in Vietnam he tried a seven-day fast. He did have a brief loss of consciousness (!) at one point because he'd lost too much salt. He hasn't repeated that mistake since. In 2015, Matt came to New Zealand, and started working at Waikato Hospital. He was routinely fasting by this point, and on a ketogenic diet. He knew there'd been some research on ketogenic diets as a treatment for the neurological disorders of Parkinson's and Alzheimer's, with promising results. He was also interested in the side effects of fasting and a ketogenic diet, not wanting to recommend something to patients until he'd tried it himself. Nowadays, Matt does a five- to seven-day fast every month.

* * *

The World Health Organization has warned that cancer is rapidly becoming a global epidemic, due to the rise of fast-food-saturated diets, sedentary lifestyles, cigarette smoking and alcohol. Cancer causes a massive burden on families and the health system. It won't be possible to treat our way out of this; prevention is preferable, more cost-effective. But how difficult will it be to change habits?

A calorie reduction of 20–40 per cent, while maintaining a normal meal pattern, has been shown to reduce cancer incidence in rodents by 75 per cent, and in rhesus monkeys by 50 per cent. It's obviously not that easy to stick to, though. Obesity is independently linked to a higher risk of many cancers. The effects of eating specific foods on cancer incidence are hard to delineate as people eat a variety of foods, and there's lots of other factors that influence cancer occurrence. However, there's a growing consensus that whole-food plant-based diets are particularly beneficial. Food writer Michael Pollan, in describing the ideal diet, says that everything he's learnt about food and health can be encapsulated in seven words: 'Eat food, not too much, mostly plants.'

Plants contain many phytonutrients, for example, carotenoids (in red, yellow or dark-green vegetables), alliums (found in garlic and onions), and polyphenols (dark chocolate – hooray!), which may work together to lower risk. Frequently eating cruciferous vegetables (cabbages, brussels sprouts – ugh, and kale) appears to decrease incidence of oesophageal and stomach cancers. The relationship between soy products and breast-cancer risk is complex and still not fully ascertained, although there is increasing evidence that moderate consumption of soy products can be protective. There's a strong link between high-fibre diets and a lower risk of colorectal cancer. Conversely, eating too much red meat, and in particular highly processed or cured meat (bacon, ham, salami), is associated with an increased risk of colorectal cancer.

Intermittent fasting (IF) involves restricting when you eat, not what you eat. Fasting has similar effects to ketogenic diets, as both methods encourage the body to burn fat because of a lack of readily available glucose stores. Fasting encourages the utilisation of endogenous (body) fat; ketogenic diets utilise exogenous (dietary) fat. Some studies on fasting show apparent benefits: improved memory and cognition, enhanced recovery after stroke, improved cholesterol, triglyceride and low-density lipoprotein levels, improvement in metabolic syndrome (which is itself a major risk factor for many diseases), reduction in obesity, and possible protection against chronic diseases such as Type II diabetes, cancers and age-related neurodegenerative conditions.

Ketogenic diets have been used for some time as a medical treatment. In children with intractable epilepsy, an older version, the classic ketogenic diet, has been used with good effect since the 1920s. It needs to be started by a medical team with close input from a trained dietitian, but it can be more effective than some seizure medications, and improve alertness and behaviour. Almost 90 per cent of the calories need to come from fats. More recently, some centres have started offering ketogenic diets to adults with epilepsy under strict criteria.

In a ketogenic diet, the dearth of calories from carbohydrates, which the body normally breaks down into glucose, stimulates the breakdown of fat stores instead. This produces ketones – acetone, beta-hydroxybutyrate – which the organs of the body, including the brain, can use as an alternative energy source. The ketosis caused by ketogenic diets or fasting, if done carefully, is generally safe. Pathological 'ketoacidosis' is a far more dangerous condition that occurs in diabetics (particularly Type I), where blood-sugar levels soar because of a lack of insulin. The body burns fat, ketones flood the system, the blood turns acidic.

There are of course potential downsides to ketogenic diets. Firstly, it can be costly to eat keto-compliant foods such as red meat, nuts and seeds. Eating too much protein can cause spikes in insulin, which defeats the purpose of the diet (Matt prefers 'adequate' rather than 'high' protein levels). It can be hard to adhere to long term, as well as being socially isolating, while some people, when they bounce off this type of diet, can regain more weight than they lost. There are restrictions on some vegetables and fruits, whole grains and low-fat dairy. Initially, keto diets can cause mood swings, tiredness, dizziness and an upset stomach – the so-called 'keto flu' – due largely to dehydration and loss of salts. These adverse effects generally improve within days to weeks of starting the diet, and by ensuring adequate fluid and salt intake.

Matt spent over four years designing a 'modified' ketogenic diet that has several advantages. It uses saturated fats such as coconut oil, which stimulates more ketones than any other kind of natural food. It's relatively affordable, not too high in protein, nor too difficult to adhere to long term. It's easily adaptable to a wide variety of cuisines and it's based on real food that stimulates the body to enter a state of physiological ketosis. He also points out that it may be beneficial to 'break' ketosis periodically. For example, when berries come into season, a glut of them may not only be delicious but also serve to create periodic insulin secretion. This 'cycling ketogenic diet' may be preferable to staying in ketosis all the time.

For decades, the advice has been to reduce overall fat intake while maintaining a moderate intake of carbohydrates. Newer evidence is emerging that it may be the combination of high fat with high carbohydrate that is deleterious to our health, not saturated fat per se. Saturated fat with a low carb load does raise low-density lipoprotein temporarily, but this appears to normalise in many people by 12 months. More significantly, perhaps, these newer keto diets also raise high-density lipoprotein (the 'good' cholesterol) and lower triglycerides.

For those wanting to do further reading, a consensus statement from the National Lipid Association is comprehensive.[19] Essentially, there are no long-term studies that properly delineate cause and effect between different sorts of diets and adverse outcomes; most studies done so far are observational. Meta-analyses of those on low-carbohydrate, high-protein, high-fat diets have shown an association with an *increase* in all-cause mortality. Matt's modified ketogenic diet advocates a low-carbohydrate, moderate- (rather than high-) protein, high-fat intake that conforms to specific parameters and that achieves a true level of physiological ketosis in the 1–2 millimoles per litre of blood range, as measured by a blood ketone monitor. Quality of life appears to improve on this, for numerous patients.

There is no one diet that will suit all people. Moreover, we have to be mindful, for example, of familial lipid disorders – ketogenic diets are not advocated for such patients as more harm than benefit can result. The overarching advice would be to discuss any potential diet carefully with a doctor experienced in diet therapy prior to starting. Nonetheless, there's increasing evidence of the efficacy of ketogenic diets and fasting on a variety of conditions: cancer, of course, but also many metabolic and neurological conditions. Fasting and ketogenic diets have been used to treat diabetes and obesity. Both appear to improve underlying insulin resistance, and reduce the hyperinsulinemic response to eating carbohydrates.[20]

Ketogenic diets can help several neurological conditions by possibly enhancing mitochondrial function. Researchers have found that mitochondrial dysfunction has an important role in many neurodegenerative disorders, such as Alzheimer's disease and Parkinson's. Matt has conducted a study on Parkinson's patients, which found that a modified ketogenic diet had a better effect on the non-motor symptoms (particularly urinary problems, pain and other sensations, fatigue, daytime sleepiness, and cognitive impairment) of Parkinson's disease than a healthy low-fat diet did.[21]

It is as yet not fully ascertained whether it is the ketones themselves, or their effects on 'anti-ageing' proteins such as sirtuins, or the effects of ketones on up-regulating mitochondrial production of ATP (adenosine triphosphate, an energy-carrying molecule found in all cells), or the increase in essential fatty acids caused by ketogenic diets, or some other method altogether, that improves function. Improvement in cognitive function has certainly been demonstrated with ketogenic diets and calorie restriction. Matt is interested in furthering research in this field. He has another study on Alzheimer's disease that is currently under review and soon to be published.

The simple beauty of glucose reduction is that it is used in many tumour-signalling pathways (cell signalling is the way cells change their activities in response to their environment). Hence, limiting glucose may help targeted drug therapies to work better. About 90 per cent of malignant cancers show an increased uptake of glucose. Some also show increased uptake of glutamine. Most show unbridled growth. When the body enters ketosis, normal cells can adapt to using ketones. Cancer cells can't. Combined with the shortage of glucose, glutamine and growth factor caused by fasting or ketosis, cancer cells become particularly susceptible to starvation and cell death. There's an increasing number of studies that show that ketogenic diets, in combination with conventional chemotherapy, can improve cancer outcomes. Periodic fasting (for two days or longer) may also be beneficial because of inducing more extreme changes in ketone, glucose, glutamine and growth-factor levels.

The effects of ketogenic diets alone, however, are at present limited to individual case studies, such as Sarona's case (which has been written up as a report in *Frontiers of Oncology*).[22] Matt Phillips is quick to emphasise that ketogenic diets in the treatment of medical conditions should be regarded as a medical intervention and administered with proper medical oversight. He is currently involved in a new study, this time involving seven glioblastoma patients. More patients continue to join and oncologists are on board. Glioblastoma is the most aggressive type of cancer originating within the brain. The median survival, with treatment, is 12 to 14 months. It is more common in the 40–60-year age group, and it is particularly difficult to treat. The tumour cells themselves are resistant to many therapies because many drugs have difficulty crossing the blood–brain barrier. The brain is easily damaged by conventional treatment and has a limited capacity to repair itself.

In the study, the patients fast for five to seven days every month, and eat a modified ketogenic diet (with plenty of 'fat bombs') on non-fasting days, in addition to their conventional treatment. Matt fasts alongside them. Sarona does the same – as tangible evidence of someone who's kicked cancer to touch, she's a beacon of hope to the others.

That silence where no sound may be

patient: Talita*; nurse: Luisa*
Caution: this chapter contains disturbing material.

Some say that pain is a universal constant. It's unavoidable, because, frankly, shit happens. Perhaps expecting bad things to happen allows us a modicum of preparation for hard times. Nonetheless, there is something particularly plangent about childhood pain. Children are not responsible for the actions of errant others, yet the pain they thus suffer can scar them for life, leave them cloven in two – an outer self that might finish school, find a job, find a partner, perform the semblances of a normal life, and an inner self that roils with secret rage, shame and guilt so fierce that the heart and mind remain trussed for years.

Given the right help and the right circumstances, pain can also mould us into people who bloom with sensitivity and empathy to the pain of others. It can make us much better at our jobs than we would have been otherwise. It is not just knowledge and skill that are the building blocks of a great nurse or doctor, but kindness, understanding, empathy. There is also a balance in maintaining professional boundaries versus divulging personal information. Yet, in the right circumstances, a medic's own story can be what a patient needs to hear in order to break their claustrophobic silence.

***

Talita* receives a routine letter asking her to come in for her first cervical-screening appointment. She books to see nurse Luisa*. Luisa oozes warmth and a non-judgemental compassion, and has a magic touch with people. She is a keen learner of facts and procedures, and she will do as much as it takes for as long as it takes for every patient.

'Have you ever been sexually active, Talita?' asks Luisa as she sets out the equipment for the test: a plastic speculum, a cervical brush and a pottle of blue liquid for the lab to perform liquid-based cytology. The test just takes a few minutes, and can be a little uncomfortable for the patient, but rarely painful. Cervical smears are recommended for any female between 25 and 70 who has ever been sexually active. Contrary to urban myth, women with female partners and transgender men (female transitioned to male) should have smears also. The human papilloma virus (HPV) that causes 99 per cent of cervical cancer works slowly, and regular smears can easily reduce the risk of this disease by up to 90 per cent. From 2023, the HPV screening test, which allows some women the option of self-testing at home and is much easier to do, will become available; this is expected to be a game-changer in the fight against cervical cancer.

The question about sexual activity is routine, and one Luisa always asks. However, 26-year-old Talita's answer is at first confusing, then alarming. 'I'm … I'm not sure,' she says.

Outside, it is a bright summer day in the South Auckland suburb of Ōtara. The heat and humidity levels are high; the air is pinguid with an oily moisture. Cloudbursts of rain are expected later that afternoon. Luisa's room looks out over a busy shopping precinct. Pedestrians throng the pavements, traffic is at a standstill. The Pasifika Festival will be held in the coming weekend, and there is a buzz in the air as school kids prepare traditional dresses for their performances.

Caught up in the busyness of the day, Luisa doesn't at first realise the subtext beneath Talita's response. 'Why is this patient being so obtuse?' she thinks. She tries to ask the question a different way, aware that there are other patients waiting, that soon she will run behind on her appointments. 'I'm sorry, I don't understand your answer, Talita. Have you ever had sex with another person?'

There is a silence that stretches for minutes, then Talita says, 'Does my uncle count?'

Luisa is struck still with horror. And then with a sinking sense of recognition. She helps Talita off the bed, sits down beside her. 'Tell me what happened, Talita, but only if you feel comfortable doing so.'

Over the next half-hour, Talita recounts her story. Sent to New Zealand from Samoa as a young girl, she was informally adopted by her mother's sister and her husband. It was a big deal to come to 'Niu Sila', with its better-recognised educational system and job opportunities. The relatives who sponsor nephews and nieces in this way are seen as providing a huge service. Talita's aunt and uncle go on to have several children. As Talita is the eldest, she is given her own room. The aunty is strict but kind.

It is when Talita turns ten that her uncle takes to lying in bed next to her after a few drinks. He touches and fondles her without her permission. He asks her if she is okay, asks her if she 'wants to play' or wants to be 'tickled'. His proximity makes her uncomfortable. Her bed becomes a cesspool of large hairy limbs and roving hands. The fourth time he comes to bed, he rapes her. Talita lies very still as this happens to her. She remembers pain. Blood. A suffocating fear.

Over the next two years, her uncle comes into her room about once a month to have sex with her. Often he is drunk; sometimes he is not. Sometimes, for protection, Talita tries to sneak into the room shared by the younger girls, but her aunt, who at this point is seemingly unaware of what her husband is up to, growls at her when she catches her sneaking around: 'We've done so much for you, even given you your own room. Why are you being so ungrateful?'

Only when Talita reaches intermediate school and observes her friends pairing up with boys their own age does she realise that what is happening to her is not normal. She becomes extremely angry and discloses the abuse to her aunt. 'Aunty was quiet for a long time,' Talita tells Luisa, 'then she said, "Don't ever tell your mother, okay?"'

Talita's aunt arranges a fa'ato'ese, an apology, from her husband. Talita is made to sit on the floor while they sit on cane chairs, and her uncle, stone-faced, apologises to her. He does not even meet her eye but stares at a spot on the wall, as if his niece were an object rather than a human being. Her aunty instructs Talita that this apology will be the end of this chapter. 'Let's now move on, let's forget about what happened,' she says. Talita is not given the opportunity to say anything at all.

'The abuse stopped after that,' Talita says. 'In fact, I still live with my aunty and uncle.'

She is calm, matter-of-fact, her face flat and devoid of emotion as she tells Luisa her story. She even laughs dismissively at one point when Luisa asks her if she is sure she is okay. 'I'm fine, I really am,' she insists. She denies the need for counselling. To this day, Talita's family do not know about the abuse, nor does Talita know if her uncle's biological daughters were similarly abused. There is just a black void, a silence, surrounding this topic in the household.

Luisa takes a deep breath. She is about to erode traditional professional boundaries by divulging her own story to Talita, but she does so hoping it will help the patient to process what happened to herself as a small, vulnerable girl.

**

Luisa was born in South Auckland, the eldest daughter of a Samoan father and a Cook Island mother. They lived in a rambling wooden house. Gardenia bushes filled the house with a sweet scent on hot summer nights, banana trees and a plot of taro were small remembrances of island life. Luisa's father was the only breadwinner, as her mother had several medical conditions that made it hard for her to work. When Luisa's younger brother was born with cerebral palsy, her mother looked after him as her health allowed.

As per Samoan custom, Luisa's father helped his brothers to come to Niu Sila. There was plenty of space in the house, while opportunities for work and a better way of life were drawcards.

The first uncle came to stay. Luisa's father was often at work and her mother was often at the hospital, so as a five-year-old she was left in the care of this uncle. Her parents assumed him to be a trustworthy adult. He sat Luisa down on a green chair and asked her, 'Do you want to play a game? Do you like tickles?' And a bolder question, as he touched himself and got her to sniff his fingers, 'Do you like this smell?'

That first uncle got a job on a farm and left Auckland before anything else could happen. When Luisa was eight, another of her dad's brothers, Uncle Lima*, came to stay. At first he was a lot of fun: he bought Luisa stuff – shoes, clothes, snacks – and he took her out on fun trips. A little while later, the dynamics changed. Lima started saying that he would only buy Luisa nice stuff if she allowed him to touch her. His room was right next to Luisa's and he struck while her parents were out. Luisa remembers encounters happening at all times of the day and night. Opportunistic episodes, an otherwise empty house, the walls of her room closing in on her. Summer or winter or spring or autumn in the streets of the neighbourhood, but always the same atmosphere inside. The duvet bunched around her ankles, her skin clammy, her heart skittering between trust and fear. Lima's fingers everywhere, sticky with guilt and pleasure. Her parents did not suspect anything – Luisa's father loved his brothers, thought the world of them. So the abuse carried on for years.

Luisa became a bully at primary school; she was a tall child and fought the boys, or she divided the girls into the 'in' crowd and the 'out' crowd. It was only as an adult that Luisa realised that being a bully at school was her way of reclaiming a little bit of control over her life. Around the age of 11, she started to feel that what was happening between herself and Uncle Lima was not normal. At the Catholic girls' school she attended, when the other girls talked about the boys they liked, boys their own age, Luisa felt ashamed that her sexual experiences were all with an older man, and a relative to boot.

Around this time, she met Joshua*, and they started dating. Joshua later admitted to being surprised at how nonchalant Luisa was about 'going all the way' with him. He became the first person whom Luisa revealed the abuse to. One night during a family get-together, while everyone else was partying in the garage and Luisa was alone in the house, Lima tried to touch her. For the first time, she said, 'Don't touch me anymore or I'll tell someone!' Joshua came over to Luisa's house for a visit and Uncle Lima found him there and beat him up in a jealous rage, pushing him against a wall that had a nail sticking out of it. The nail snagged against the back of 13-year-old Joshua's scalp. Lima later berated Luisa: 'How could you do this to me?' A man in his thirties; the jilted lover.

With Joshua now in Luisa's life, Lima finally left her alone. She started spending more and more time at Joshua's house, with the blessing of Joshua's parents, but Luisa's father was not happy, and said, 'Why are you embarrassing us like this?' She was 18 years old. She told him everything that had happened between herself and his two brothers. Her dad grabbed his can of beer, was silent for some time, then finally said, 'Don't tell your mum.'

That may have been it, like it was for patient Talita. However, in the typical manner of how abusive or overtly sexualised behaviour can spread from person to person, a cousin who Luisa had played with, sexually, when they were both younger, was caught having sex with someone else. He blurted out that Luisa introduced him to this behaviour. A family meeting was called. Luisa's father slapped her in front of everyone as a public display of punishment. 'What have you done?' he thundered. She broke down crying and revealed the abuse she had suffered at the hands of her uncles. Uncle Lima was later made to apologise to Luisa's parents, but not to Luisa herself. Luisa's mother was asked to forgive Lima, and then to just move on, to 'just forget about it'.

Luisa was left feeling like she was the guilty one. She stayed away from her father's family for years. She married Joshua, and they had two kids. She admits these days to watching her own daughter like a hawk; only close relatives can look after her, and she explicitly checks that no one is touching her daughter inappropriately. Lots of questions are directed at this small, precious child.

Then, at a family funeral, adult Luisa came face to face with Uncle Lima. She accosted him, told him how his sexual abuse affected her. He apologised properly this time, and disclosed his own abuse as a ten-year-old back in Samoa. This apology and revelation brought a small degree of understanding. But the childhood abuse left Luisa with a hugely depleted sense of self-esteem, and at the age of 28, she finally undertook counselling for two years, then art therapy. The counselling helped, but the art therapy in particular has been excellent for her. 'It brings out my inner child, and with that comes so much peace and healing. I love it.'

***

Traumatic abuse is sadly not uncommon and it spans the spectrum of ethnicities. There are certain factors that make some groups of New Zealanders more vulnerable to this form of violence, however. Statistics in New Zealand echo those in other countries.

They show that one in three girls may be sexually abused before they turn 16 years old. The figure is slightly lower for young boys – one in seven may be sexually abused prior to adulthood – but still significant, traumatic and impactful. Up to 90 per cent of the abuse will be perpetrated by someone known to the victim, usually a male family member. Seventy per cent of the time, genital contact will be involved; for 50 per cent of victims, the abuse can occur on multiple occasions. Young people are at the highest risk of being sexually assaulted. Those in the 16–24 age group are four times more likely to be assaulted than any other group. Those with physical or other disabilities are also more vulnerable.

While sexual violence is not restricted to certain ethnic groups, complex factors perpetuate its existence in some cohorts, from childhood through to adulthood. A paper in 2019 by Dr Rachel Simon-Kumar, of the School of Population Health at the University of Auckland, found that more than one in two Māori women reported past or current sexual violence; Asian women reported such violence the least, at one in ten; prevalence rates in Pasifika and Pākehā were roughly equivalent to each other, at one in three.[23]

The rate of substantive childhood abuse in Māori children under seventeen is almost twice the rate in non-Māori children in the same age bracket. Socio-economic disadvantages such as unemployment, poor housing and poverty are linked in numerous studies to these higher rates of childhood abuse. Many studies have also shown that strong affiliations with a Māori cultural identity, and with it wider whānau relationships and tikanga, can have a protective factor against child abuse, possibly because of the increased relational buffering and self-esteem these things provide.

As always, there are multiple factors feeding in to these statistics. One important point to note is that sexual violence is almost certainly under-reported across the societal spectrum. This is especially true for Asian communities, where there is a strong drive to 'save face' and prevent shame. Some cultures hold women responsible for sexual violence, especially when female purity or virginity is highly prized, and this is something that both Luisa and Talita experienced. Again, this leads to under-reporting of abuse.

Migration has its effects. For some men coming from traditionally male-dominated cultures, migration can mean a loss of mana or status, a perceived loss of authority and the uncertainty of unemployment. All of these things can trigger sexual or domestic violence. Minority ethnic women can end up in low-paying or menial jobs, which can perpetuate their inability to escape abuse. Migrants may not be aware of their rights under law. There may be a lack of trust in officials such as police, hospital doctors or social workers, who may be perceived as racist – there is certainly a tendency by some in authority to frame gender violence as a 'normal' attribute of a particular minority or cultural group rather than as a problem across cultures. This stigma further impedes victims from seeking help.

Abuse of a young child leaves permanent scars on their psyche, unless therapeutic interventions are carried out. Nurse

Luisa knows this first-hand: the art therapy, in particular, has been life-changing for her. Until she started therapy, she carried so much guilt and self-blame for her childhood abuse. But it would seem that Talita is, at the very least, still stuck in denial, stricken by silence. Although she listened as Luisa shared her story that day, she did not seem to change her stoic attitude. Luisa helped direct Talita towards resources that could help, for example, options such as funded counselling through ACC.

It can be hard for some victims to recognise that what happened to them was 'abuse'. Especially if it happens insidiously, with grooming and initial innocuous activities, doubt can exist in the victim's mind as to their own culpability: did I encourage this? Was it my fault? The average victim takes 24 years to reveal their childhood trauma. The power of self-blame is immense. Some people may never disclose their history of abuse; some may only do so in their eighties or nineties. Some children who try to report abuse are silenced, minimised or dismissed. They may even be punished, further stamping them with a sense of blame.

Male victims are much less likely to disclose abuse. As most perpetrators are male, young boys can be left confused and ashamed about their own sexuality. Disclosure can lead to discrimination and humiliation in cultures where men are expected to be strong and not cry. There is also a degree of fear around male victims of childhood sexual abuse becoming perpetrators themselves when they are older. Many studies have found this to be true in only a minority of male sex offenders (around the 25 per cent mark), but the myth of a victim-to-perpetrator cycle persists. There are some factors that can make male victims of sexual abuse more likely to become perpetrators themselves, including more severe abuse, sexual abuse committed by a woman, limited emotional support from family and friends, and adjustment difficulties or mental-health problems in childhood and adolescence.

The World Health Organization recognises the existence of complex post-traumatic stress disorder, and it is thought that many survivors of childhood abuse suffer from this. It differs from other forms of PTSD because sufferers can have a more pervasive and rigid negative belief about themselves. Feelings of shame and inadequacy can hold survivors of abuse back from fully participating in school or work. Some show a significant increase in mood disorders and suicide attempts (up to one in five survivors), and can fall into addictive behaviours later in life. Many have difficulties with interpersonal relationships, with some avoiding sexual intimacy altogether, while others gravitate towards sexual promiscuity.

Childhood abuse can lead to poorer physical health – an increase in heart disease and cancer, among other things – and a shorter life span due to the effects of chronic stress. There can be a two-fold increase in susceptibility to later physical violence as adult survivors become vulnerable to predators in their desperation to be loved. There are also increased incidences of 'social problems' such as teenage pregnancy, single parenting and lifetime low-socioeconomic status. These statistics are a testament to the interplay of emotion, physiology, environment and genetics as underlying factors in all human behaviour, whether healthy or maladaptive.

Childhood sexual abuse sits alongside other adverse childhood experiences, such as physical abuse and neglect, which create a toxic constellation of health issues. So often we try to control the symptoms, the drink and drug use, the depression and so on, without asking *why* a person is behaving as they are. However, it's not all bad news. Survivors can thrive, can heal, can grow with the right input. Children and adults do not have to be irredeemably damaged for life.

Society and our communities can help. It's incredibly important to take disclosure seriously – for many victims, not being believed when they finally pluck up the courage can be a rejection so immense that it is as, or more, traumatic than the original abuse. Specialist services, once contacted, should intervene early to provide a safe, nurturing environment that allows healing and prevents future abuse. Adults who seek counselling are far better equipped to heal from their experiences. A big part of the therapeutic process is to take back the power of shame and blame and, instead, speak out so that other victims may also come forward. Good therapy can help victims replace the negative self-talk and poor self-esteem with recognition, acceptance and self-love.

Legal repercussions for perpetrators are still infuriatingly light. Only ten out of 100 sexual-abuse crimes are reported in New Zealand (this figure must, in reality, be even lower, as the true prevalence of this societal evil is probably higher than what is reported). Of those ten, only three will make it to court, and in only one out of those 100 cases will the perpetrator be prosecuted.

In Talita's case, there is still much that is hidden – possibly a sense of shame, a sense of denial. It is hard to tell. By her own account, she has never had the chance to tell her uncle how the abuse affected her, she has only received a superficial apology, and was then instructed to put it all behind her. She has never had counselling, and denies she needs this.

For Luisa, her childhood trauma has fundamentally shaped both her character and her career path. She is a ceaseless advocate for the rights of women and girls. She is outspoken on the effects of childhood and domestic abuse, particularly in her own community. Luisa has undertaken a domestic violence course for medical professionals run by Shine Women's Refuge, so that she can further help needy patients who are not always willing to divulge their abuse or seek help.

'I want to speak out. In Pasifika culture, as in many other cultures, the victim may feel like the guilty one. I think underneath Talita's denial lies a lot of unresolved hurt, guilt and shame. Meeting Talita has made me all the more determined to help. I want patients like her to be able to say, "I was abused, and it was not my fault. I survived, and I will get my life back."'

The changing face of general practice

patient: Fran*; GP: Dr Leonard Prior*

General practice in New Zealand has transformed significantly over the last four decades. Dr Leonard (Len) Prior* remembers lots of patient encounters, both harrowing and entertaining, including politicians, rugby players and others who have graced his waiting rooms in South Auckland in order to get checked over and have 'a hearty yarn with Len'. But there's one patient in particular whose story Len finds hard to forget. It was an obstetric emergency in the summer of 1981 that became fraught with hospital politics, the fallout of which led to significant, ongoing changes in Len's job.

***

202

When Len's patient Fran* turns up to the delivery suite at Middlemore Hospital in labour, the staff ring him to come in, as he is her designated GP obstetrician (GPO). Although Len works primarily in his own general practice clinic in South Auckland, he has a contract with the health board to make use of rooms in the delivery suite for pregnant patients. Like many of his GP colleagues at this time, he manages pregnant patients from conception through to delivery. It's one of the most meaningful parts of his job. A 'cradle to the grave' philosophy of medicine that is built on a unique, and sometimes life-long, relationship.

Friday-afternoon traffic is fitful as Len finishes his GP clinic and drives to the hospital. He knows he will be there for hours tonight, possibly for most of the weekend – he'll have to get a greasy meal from the hospital cafeteria later. The delivery suite is busy. Some of the other patients also have GPOs attending to them; Len knows these colleagues well. Others have midwives or obstetricians. Len grabs a cup of coffee and heads off to find Fran.

Fran is in her thirties. This is her second pregnancy, her first full-term birth. Her first pregnancy, to a previous partner, ended in a late miscarriage. Fran's partner is with her. He's given a supply of cold flannels to place on her forehead as the need arises. He is also Len's patient; blunt and at times assertive. He paces up and down, glares at Len, paces some more. This is unnerving for Len.

At first, Fran is calm enough. She's ready for this; she's been to her antenatal classes and feels prepped. The contractions come and go, time slips by. But as the hours stretch on and on, and her labour becomes obstructed, Fran's discomfort and frustration mount. Len assesses Fran with a cardiotocograph (CTG), a machine that monitors the foetal heart and uterine contractions. The CTG has a flat belt that is strapped to Fran's abdomen, and inside this belt are two disc-shaped transducers that use an ultrasound called a Doppler to pick up the rate at which Fran's baby's heart is beating, and the strength of the uterine contractions. It is a safe and noninvasive method of monitoring foetal well-being. A normal foetal heart rate sits at 110–160 beats per minute, which is much higher than an adult's. As the uterus contracts, the foetal heart rate should vary a little. If it doesn't, or if it is too high or too low, it may indicate a problem.

A CTG is not always needed for all deliveries, particularly if the pregnancy has been low risk, but if there is evidence of an issue, such as maternal fever or high blood pressure, or if there is evidence of foetal distress, then it can be used to monitor the health of the baby. Of note, even healthy pregnancies can end up with unforeseen complications during labour and delivery, such as a haemorrhage. The difference between life and death, or between life and severe complications, can be measured in minutes.

The CTG shows that Fran is in early labour, with contractions lasting 30 seconds occurring every 15 minutes or so. The action of the uterus contracting shortens and widens the cervix, the doughnut-shaped muscle at the lower end of the womb. Normally the cervix is only about 2–3 centimetres long, and a few centimetres wide. Prior to delivery, the cervix acts as the plug that keeps the baby in, and the outside world (with its attendant cast of microbes) out. As labour starts, various hormones are released, which change the collagen structure in the cervix. The cervix transforms from a firmish plug into a super-stretchy entity. The cervical os (the 'hole' in the middle of the doughnut that connects the vagina to the uterus) is normally less than 8 millimetres wide. An average full-term infant head is roughly 94 millimetres across, and the cervix has to stretch to accommodate this.

Fran is not aware of all the changes going on inside her body. Mostly what she feels is discomfort and pressure, and thirst, tiredness and a desire to sleep. Fran's cervix has dilated to 3 centimetres when Len examines her. She is ready to enter the active labour phase, where contractions will become stronger and more regular, and where the cervix will continue to stretch and dilate. Len breaks Fran's membranes (the fluid-filled amniotic sac that has kept the baby separate from the outside world for the last nine months). This rupture of membranes, or 'breaking the waters', usually happens naturally. It is important for this to occur so that Fran can move into the active phase.

When the waters break on this occasion, however, what rushes out is not just straw-coloured amniotic fluid but thick olive-green meconium. Meconium is the first bowel output of many mammals. It is not like normal faeces, composed as it is of bile, mucus, amniotic fluid, vernix (the greasy whitish substance that coats a newborn's skin), pancreatic juices, and other substances ingested by the infant in utero. Meconium is odourless but very thick and sticky, almost tar-like. Normally it should pass within

24 hours of birth, but sometimes, as in Fran's case, the baby may pass meconium while still inside the womb. This can be a sign of foetal distress. It can also be passed by post-date babies. Left untreated, it can lead to meconium aspiration syndrome, where the thick stuff ends up in the baby's lungs, causing inflammation and infection.

But Fran's baby is a good size and is not distressed. The CTG shows a good foetal heart rate with a good degree of variability. Len inserts a foetal scalp electrode, via Fran's vagina, onto the baby's scalp to better monitor his or her heartbeat. He also starts Fran on a syntocinon infusion. Syntocinon is a synthetic form of the naturally occurring hormone oxytocin and can help augment labour by increasing the contractility of the uterus, thus speeding up the process. Naturally occurring oxytocin is produced by the hypothalamus gland in the brain. It is released during labour to help with contractions, and also released in the postpartum period during breast-feeding, helping to initiate maternal bonding with the infant. Its release in other settings, such as during sexual intercourse or in social settings, helps us to bond with our partners or with platonic members of our social groups. The proverbial 'rush of affection' we feel for others.

The cervix dilates about 1 centimetre per hour during the active labour phase. Fran starts to experience stronger contractions, lasting about a minute and occurring every three to five minutes. There is an ache in her lower back and painful contractions radiating to her stomach area. She says she feels like her insides are being stretched, pulled, twisted. There's a surge of hormones and inflammatory proteins coursing through her veins that are working in tandem to help her deliver her baby. She gets pain relief via an intravenous line. Her partner massages her shoulders and her back but he is tired and fractious himself. He flops back on a chair for a rest. This labour is a marathon. It is now the early hours of Saturday morning. The sun peeps through the hospital windows, but everyone in the room is too fatigued to feel cheered. Len pops out for a quick breather, grabs another cup of coffee.

Fran's cervix dilates to 8 centimetres and then stubbornly refuses to dilate any further. The baby's head isn't descending into her pelvis, isn't engaging. Time marches on. Len updates Fran on the lack of progress. She feels frustrated. Something needs to give.

The baby's heart rate starts to show dips to a rate of 80, lasting a few seconds only, then coming back to baseline. Then the foetal heart rate starts to show variable decelerations, down to 60 beats per minute, rising back up to baseline but only slowly. A stab of alarm cuts through the tired fug in Len's head. These decelerations indicate the baby is getting tired. Once this is noted, it is important to aim for an emergency caesarean section within ten minutes. Len examines Fran once more; her cervix is still only 8 centimetres. 'Time to change tack,' he thinks. He turns off the syntocinon infusion.

'Fran, I think your baby's getting dangerously tired,' Len says. 'I'll need to hand you over to the on-call obstetrician for a C-section asap.'

Fran glares at Len, at her partner, then back at Len. She shakes her head vehemently. 'No, I don't want that consultant anywhere near my baby!' she shouts. As she struggles up from the hospital bed, the swell of her pregnant abdomen looms between herself and Len. Another labour contraction makes her lie down again, and she huffs until it passes, the skin on her belly tight. She grabs hold of Len's arm. 'I am NOT going to that man, Len. Don't you bloody hand me over to him!' Fran works at Middlemore as a theatre nurse and she knows the on-call obstetrician all too well. He has an infamous reputation. Despite her fatigue, despite the fact that this delivery now needs urgent obstetric intervention, she is resolute.

Len leaves the room. He is trying not to panic, trying to think his way out of this situation. In the corridor, he bumps into another obstetrician – a good friend, a professor of obstetrics – who is not on call but fortuitously is in the hospital that morning doing his own rounds.

'I need help,' Len says, explaining his predicament. The professor moves quickly. He asks Len if he wants to do the C-section himself; he knows that Len has done plenty of these during his time as an obstetric registrar, however, Len's contract with Middlemore stipulates that patients in Fran's circumstances must be handed over for further management. Also, the situation has become tense, and Len is exhausted. He asks the obstetrician to go ahead without him. Fran's baby is born shortly afterwards via a C-section, and comes out kicking and screaming. Len will see the baby later, in his general practice clinic, for the baby's six-week immunisations.

For now, Len leaves Middlemore and drives home. He has been up all night, and is looking forward to bed. However, something sparks a light in his sleep-deprived mind. He remembers he is supposed to be on call for the Saturday morning clinic at his own general practice. Len groans. There is no option but to turn around and drive there. After all, the keys are in his pocket. When he arrives, the carpark is full of patients waiting to be seen. Len gets home at 11 pm on Saturday night.

One week later, Len gets an official letter of complaint from the hospital. The letter outlines that Dr Leonard Prior did not hand over the patient to the appropriate on-call member of staff. Fran's case, and the exhaustion of juggling a busy GP clinic with obstetric cases that can last for hours and hours, conspire to encourage Len to stop being a GP obstetrician, even though delivering babies is one of the most satisfying aspects of his job.

***

Len's father fought in World War II before Len was born. When he returned, he was given a financial incentive to settle in South Auckland. The Land Settlement Board passed legislation allowing some ex-servicemen access to Crown land, with rehabilitation loans at low rates of interest. So Len's father purchased a rambling old homestead in Manurewa. He married Len's mother in 1949; she was from Wanganui farming stock. Self-reportedly 'hopeless at school', she later went to Elam School of Fine Arts. Her own father was a World War I veteran. He killed himself when she was just 17 years old.

Len grew up surrounded by acres of green farmland. 'Back then Manurewa was just a village. It was green all the way from Puhinui Road to Russell Road.' Down the main street there was a village store that sold essentials: tubes of toothpaste (without fluoride – this got added later, in the 1960s), blocks of butter, tall glass bottles of milk, bins of flour with a metal scoop. The Pākehā butcher hung carcasses in his coolstore, with sawdust on the floor to soak up blood. A New Zealand Chinese family ran the local greengrocers; their shelves groaned with vibrant fresh produce. Sacks of dirt-crusted potatoes, tomatoes saturated with sunshine. Len rode his bike everywhere. He went to a small Catholic school with only 13 children in his class, and had a happy childhood, until the age of ten when he became aware of parental conflict. His father's heavy drinking started to seep out during daylight hours. Looking back, Len realises his father had post-traumatic stress disorder. Many servicemen from that era returned with symptoms of psychological distress, but there was no recognition or treatment available for this. Instead, they were advised to 'man up' and get on with life, to forget about the 'monstrous anger of the guns' and the 'stuttering rifles' rapid rattle'.[24]

His parents eventually separated and his father died of alcoholic cardiomyopathy when Len was just 23. His mother worked hard as an illustrator of fashion garments for major stores such as Smith & Caughey's and Milne & Choyce. The garments were delivered to her studio, where she sketched till the early hours of the morning. Len applied for medical school, because 'that's where the top brains went in those days'. Despite being from a poor, small school, he got in. He trained in Auckland, did his elective in Canada, came home, and met and married his wife. Len did a stint in obstetrics, and his seniors were keen for him to pursue this as a career.

He initially wanted to travel first before beginning a family, but this plan changed when his wife's father got untreatable bowel cancer, and so he did a locum in general practice instead in South Auckland, and ended up buying into the practice, where he has worked ever since. 'General practice has really suited my personality. Although perhaps I would have made more money if I'd trained as a hospital specialist, being a GP has given me a wonderful life. I have a strong marriage, three wonderful kids, and I feel like I've achieved some things during my time in this clinic.'

Len is looking forward to retirement, despite some ongoing physical issues. He's definitely looking forward to not getting up early every morning to go to work. When I interview Len, he has been a GP for over 40 years. He's incredibly hard-working, and churns through more patient appointments than younger colleagues. His patients adore him; his retirement will be a blow to hundreds of people. If it were not for health issues, he may have kept working into his seventies.

* * *

General practice in New Zealand has changed a lot since Len started. He says it is better in some ways: the days of being on call almost 24 hours a day, seven days a week, were unsustainable. Weekends were a particular nightmare, as the doctor could be called out anytime between Friday afternoon and Monday morning. Notably, this is still the situation for some rural GPs. When Len and his colleagues first opened their clinic in 1974, nurses from the DHB were seconded there, and medical supplies were provided free by the DHB. A surgeon, a gynaecologist and an ophthalmologist all ran free clinics using different rooms in the practice. The government funding per patient consult was about $1.25; the patient was charged up to five dollars.

All patient notes were handwritten onto small cards that were stored alphabetically. Brevity was of the essence, although legibility could be poor – one thing that hasn't changed since the time of Hippocrates is a doctor's handwriting. Computerisation of notes is probably the biggest improvement that Len has encountered. He also acknowledges that the doctor–patient relationship in the 'bad old days' definitely tended towards the patriarchal. 'It was a case of "take these pills, dear" rather than "would you like to take these pills and here's what they might do to you". We did not learn how to listen to people's emotions at medical school. There's a lot more of that being taught now.'

The role of the GP obstetrician has certainly declined in many Western countries in the last 30 years. A paper by Otago University found this was due in part to the difficulties of juggling high clinical workloads, poor remuneration, higher costs of malpractice insurance, and the difficulty of maintaining skills.[25] Since the 1950s, social movements in New Zealand and around the world have advocated for removing the medical profession's control of childbirth. In the 1980s, midwives campaigned to be allowed to deliver babies without a doctor being present. The Nurses Amendment Act of 1990 recognised midwives as autonomous health professionals. Until 1996, when a new funding model eventuated, about half of all women giving birth had a GP obstetrician handling their care; in recent years, this figure has dropped to 2–3 per cent or less. There are still some GPOs practising, particularly rurally, and they cite job satisfaction as a major motivation.

Fran's case was what caused Len to stop doing obstetrics, and after the political fallout from it, he terminated his contract with the delivery suite. Although he continued to look after pregnant patients and their babies, Len still misses the joy of delivering babies. Fran acknowledged afterwards that she had put Len in an impossible bind at the time.

There's a bunch of other things that have changed too. In the 1970s, the hospital ran clinics for high-blood-pressure and chronic-illness patients. There has been a shift in care of these issues to GPs. In terms of lifestyle-related illnesses, diabetes was a rare entity in the 1970s, but from the 1980s onwards, with both an increase in immigration and an increased availability of fast food and takeaways, obesity mushroomed, and New Zealand adults are now the third most obese in the OECD. Diabetes affects 6 per cent of the population. Cardiovascular disease kills one in three.

Much of the burden of chronic-care management now rests with GPs. General practice used to be reactive – the proverbial ambulance at the bottom of the cliff – albeit with long-term relational management. Now it's more proactive, seeking to identify and prevent illness from happening. Many GPs nowadays have special interests and secondary-level skills in various fields, such as palliative care, obstetrics, musculoskeletal medicine, addiction care, dermoscopy and mental health.

But it would be fair to say general practice in New Zealand is not in a good state. With regard to funding, the 2000s saw the creation of primary health organisations (PHOs) in an attempt to increase access to primary care. There are now 30 PHOs in existence. This is an absurd balkanisation of services for such a small country. There are also 20 district health boards to add to the complexity. DHBs theoretically should fund all health services in their districts; however, funding is heavily weighted towards hospitals rather than primary care. The previous fee-for-service system moved to a capitated funding system in the 2000s, where each enrolled patient received funding per head (per capita), rather than the practice being funded for each visit the patient makes. It is increasingly recognised that the capitation model is outdated and needs to be rejigged to take into account complex patient factors, such as health status, age, gender, income, geographic access and ethnicity.

Practices operate as small to medium businesses, yet unlike other privately run businesses, income is strictly controlled. Rigidly capped capitation payments lead to chronic underfunding; meanwhile, costs continue to escalate. The Covid-19 pandemic cast a clear light on how financially vulnerable many general practices are. GPs are doing increasing amounts of paperwork during lunchbreaks or evenings, without being paid for this non-clinical time, whereas hospital counterparts are. There are also issues with the physician workforce itself: a recent survey carried out by the GP College (The Royal New Zealand College of General Practitioners) shows that the average age of a GP is 50, and that one-third plan to retire in the next five years.

The above constraints are unfortunate. There is much advantage to be had in a robust general practice sector: relational, trust-based medicine practised over the course of multiple consults by a health professional who is well known to the patient is in a different league to transactional, momentary health encounters. Excellent primary healthcare can lead to better population health. A study in the *Journal of the American Medical Association* showed that primary care was associated with more high-value care, more utilisation of preventative health measures and better outcomes.[26] Such data doesn't exist here, due to geographical and informational fragmentation caused by the fact that there is poor to little sharing of medical information between different DHBs.

In April 2021, in response to the Health and Disability System Report (HDSR), Minister of Health Andrew Little announced the intention to make widespread changes to New Zealand's health sector. Instead of multiple DHBs, there will now be one single Crown entity, Health New Zealand. This will have four regional divisions. A new Māori Health Authority will monitor and seek to improve Māori health. The HDSR found that beefing up primary healthcare would potentially lead to the most improvement in the health of New Zealanders – welcome confirmation of what many general practitioners have long believed to be true. The proposed changes, if done thoroughly and with the explicit involvement of key players, could remove many barriers to integrated, equitable healthcare across the nation.

***

Fran implicitly trusted Len, and leaned hard on him during her tense delivery. It was a trust built on years of relationship. Len continued to look after her and her family as her little boy grew up – even up to when he started his own family. Truly generational care. As with all his patients, Len strove to provide exemplary holistic care. He went the extra mile, did all those intangible things that cannot be measured by concrete parameters but that tell a patient and their whānau that someone has their back. Who can put a price on that?

Going home

patient: Tom*; GP: Dr Jason Tuhoe
Information also from Tom's wife.

Tom* is a Pākehā man in his thirties. Dr Jason Tuhoe is a hard-working rural GP based in a smallish town. Because the very nature of a small town tends to blur traditional medic–patient boundaries, his patients are friends, neighbours, relatives, the local police. Hence Jason knows Tom and his wife well.

Jason asks Tom to come in for a face-to-face consult. The discussion that he has to have today can't be done over the phone. It's the sort of conversation that fills most doctors with dread. Jason has always got on so well with Tom; this particular medic–patient relationship has been strutted over the years with easy banter and commonalities. They are both around the same age and stage in life – married with young kids. These similarities cast a chill on Jason when Tom falls ill. When you see someone as young as yourself become unexpectedly sick, you feel vulnerable. And you feel guilty as hell that you are still healthy and enjoying a normal life.

Tom is a generous, capable sort. He works as a builder. Fit and healthy, with a smattering of freckles on his cheeks and strong forearms corded with veins, he's a jack of all trades. On weekends he likes to do a bit of DIY – drilling holes in walls, assembling a deck. Recently, he's been driving a Bobcat on a building site. One day, he injures his back while lifting and cutting logs, slicing pine into rough-hewn planks, stacking them in piles. When a stack of planks slips and Tom grabs at them, he wrenches his back.

The pain in his back niggles on and on. A month passes. Then another month. Tom hopes it will get better but it gets worse instead, a crab-like pain that grabs Tom with both pincers and squeezes hard. Won't let him sleep. Makes him hold his breath in the middle of the night so he doesn't yell and wake his wife up. He can't get comfortable, whether he sits or stands or lies down. He starts to get abdominal pains also. Odd cramps here and there. As if, every so often, that malicious crab reaches a claw deep inside and pinches soft, sensitive tissue without mercy.

Finally, Tom comes in for a check-up with Jason. Any back pain that lasts longer than a month, especially with attendant night-time pain, warrants imaging, so Jason sends Tom for a routine X-ray of his lumbar spine, funded by ACC. The images show numerous black holes, peppered like gunshot, all through what should be whitish bone in Tom's lumbar spine. He's also got a crush fracture at L3, the probable cause of his persistent pain. These osteolytic lesions (essentially, holes in the bone) are often caused by cancers seeding through the bloodstream into bone. As the lytic lesions enlarge, the weakened vertebral bone collapses, leading to a crush fracture. This is immensely painful.

Cancer is not at the top of the diagnostic list at this stage. Not when Tom is only 33 years old. There are other possible causes of these lesions. Atypical haemangiomas. Aneurysmal bone cysts. Benign osteoid osteomas. However, metastatic lesions from multiple myeloma, melanoma, or lung, gastrointestinal or renal cancer, need to be excluded. Jason orders an MRI via the on-call radiologist to help provide a definitive diagnosis.

An MRI involves lying on a plinth inside a cylindrical noisy tube. It takes detailed scans using magnetic fields and radio waves to delineate the distribution of water and fat in our bodies, and is excellent for looking at torn muscles and broken bones. They take much longer than CT scans, and are not amenable to those who suffer from claustrophobia or who have vital and immovable bits of metal implanted in their bodies. On this occasion, the MRI shows suspicious lesions on Tom's lumbar spine and in his liver, and a large tumour in his rectum, with nearby enlarged nodes. The prognosis is not good. It looks like metastatic cancer, which has clearly spread to Tom's bones, liver and lymph nodes. The liver is a common site for colon cancer spread, via the portal vein, which drains blood from the gut to the liver and spleen.

Jason immediately asks Tom and his wife to come in. When he tells them the results of the scan, as gently as he can, the usually garrulous Tom is shocked into silence. He stares at the floor. Minutes pass. Then he looks at Jason. 'But there must be some mistake, Jason. Surely?'

Further questioning reveals that in fact Tom has been having altered bowel motions for some months, has had weight loss, even some intermittent rectal bleeding. Tom had put the bleeding down to long-standing haemorrhoids, and the weight loss to being so busy lately he wasn't eating properly.

A subsequent urgent colonoscopy and biopsy confirm rectal adenocarcinoma. Tom switches from shock to anger. He is so young. He feels life has dealt him a cruel and grossly unfair hand. He wants to be around for his children as they grow up. He wants to be a good husband to his wife. 'Till death do us part' was not supposed to eventuate so early in married life. 'Why me?' he asks Jason, over and over. He seesaws between hope of a miraculous cure and a suffocating despair.

This meeting marks a new phase in the doctor–patient relationship. Dr Jason Tuhoe has long held a special interest in palliative care. It is a useful adjunctive skill for a rural GP to have; there are not enough hospices and palliative-care specialists to cover all areas of New Zealand. However, Jason has never had to use his expertise to look after a patient as young as Tom before. There are tears, from Tom and his wife, from Jason. There is Tom's refusal, over the next two years, to acknowledge that he is dying. There is Jason's ongoing tussle with misplaced guilt, his struggle to maintain clinical objectivity.

***

How did Tom develop what is usually thought of as an older person's disease? Something in Tom's family history did increase his risk. Tom's mother has Lynch syndrome – hereditary non-polyposis colorectal cancer (HNPCC), an inherited cancer syndrome associated with a genetic predisposition to different types of cancer. Lynch syndrome patients have a significantly increased risk of developing colorectal cancer under the age of 50. There is also an increased risk of developing other cancers, such as endometrial, stomach, breast, prostate or liver cancer. Medically, Lynch syndrome is suspected when clusters of different cancers occur in a family. Estimates suggest as many as one in every 300 people may be carriers. Tom was previously tested for Lynch syndrome, and cleared, however, he may have had a different genetic variant to his mother, one that wasn't able to be picked up with testing.

Worldwide, colorectal cancer is the second-leading cause of cancer death. Diets high in red and processed meats but low in fibre, high alcohol intake, cigarette smoking, obesity, sedentary lifestyles – these are all associated with increased rates. Researchers are also looking into links between the gut biome and the onset of colorectal cancer, and whether using antibiotics has any bearing on this.

New Zealand has one of the highest rates of bowel cancer in the world. It is our second-highest cause of death from cancer. About 3000 New Zealanders are diagnosed with it annually (Ministry of Health); about 1200 people die every year from it. About a quarter of patients are only diagnosed when they turn up with significant symptoms, late in the course of their disease. A study in 2018 showed Māori and Pasifika patients have worse outcomes.[27] Another study, published in *The Lancet*,[28] noted a small but worrying increase in the incidence of colorectal cancers in those under 50. New Zealand was one of the countries studied. Rates of colon cancer over a ten-year period in our under-50s were up by 2.9 per cent. They were up by similar amounts in Australia and Denmark, while in the UK, the rates in this age group were up by 1.8 per cent. The absolute risk of colorectal cancer in this age group remains low, though, at fewer than five cases per 100,000.

Patients in New Zealand aged 60 to 74 get free screening with a faecal immunochemical test (FIT). Out of 1000 tests, 50 people will have a positive test; 35 of these will have polyps on colonoscopy; three or four will be found to have bowel cancer. It's different for younger patients like Tom, however. Most cases in younger patients are sporadic rather than inherited. They don't always qualify for a colonoscopy, unless they have a strong family history. Because Tom falls into the 'high risk' category, due to the family history of HNPCC, he would have been eligible for a colonoscopy from the age of 25 – if he'd come to his GP with at least a six-week history of altered bowel habit or unexplained rectal bleeding. It just never crossed his mind that his symptoms were such a sinister portent.

Tom grudgingly submits to treatment at Waikato Hospital's oncology department. The biopsy result from his rectal tumour helps to guide the type of chemotherapy that he receives. Most chemo drugs for bowel cancer are publicly funded for New Zealand patients. Immunotherapy drugs, which specifically target the abnormal mutations in cancer cells by mimicking or modulating the patient's immune system, can be used as an adjunct to traditional chemotherapy to boost treatment, but these 'targeted' therapies are not publicly funded. If the oncologist feels that they could be pursued (based on the biopsy results), the patient could choose to pay for these.

Tom and his wife opt for traditional chemotherapy initially. The cost of targeted therapies is too high for this young family to contemplate. The treatment is palliative rather than curative; medics are unable to cure cancer that has spread so widely. However, treatment can extend life and help alleviate some of the tumour symptoms. Balanced against this will be side effects from the treatment itself. Side effects usually resolve with time, once each cycle of chemotherapy finishes, but they are debilitating – tiredness, diarrhoea, a sore mouth, ulcers, hair loss, numb fingers and toes.

Surgery is discussed with Tom, to be offered on a palliative basis to relieve symptoms if the tumour obstructs his gut, for example. Radiotherapy is also offered. This will be given over five to six weeks in order to help shrink the rectal cancer, reduce obstructive symptoms and improve quality of life. But it, too, brings side effects of tiredness, broken skin, diarrhoea, nausea.

Tom suffers with excruciating pain from the metastatic lesions in his back. The malicious crab is clawing flesh and bone from within. The constant pain dims his smile and his usually chirpy can-do outlook. It is hard for his wife to watch her husband shrink before her eyes. Tom has nausea and fatigue during the chemotherapy cycles; his hair falls out. It is a time of tiredness and misery. His children are too young to understand why their dad doesn't want to do stuff with them anymore.

Jason walks alongside Tom, encouraging him, fielding his questions, advocating for him. The different therapies do not cure the cancer, but they give Tom two precious years of life post-diagnosis.

As a Christian, Tom doesn't appear to struggle with his faith during this ordeal, even though loss of faith or purpose can be a common response to a terminal diagnosis. Instead, his faith gives him a modicum of understanding, a structure to the way he responds to his diagnosis, a strong belief that death will not be the end but a homecoming. He tries to maintain a positive outlook despite the ongoing tread of disease. He posts encouraging messages on Facebook: 'I'm being invited to the House of the Lord,' he writes. 'Normally when it is time to leave someone's house, they don't fill up your glass. But in this House, my glass is always overflowing.'

He decides to tick some things off his bucket list, so he chooses to go to India. The oncologists are hesitant about him flying so far away while he is unwell, but Tom is determined to go. 'If not now, when?' he reasons. The trip is full of colour, noise, mounds of spices in open-air markets, chaotic traffic, ancient architecture. It does a world of good for his mood. A little bit of the old Tom resurfaces – until he has to cut short the trip and fly back home when the pain becomes unbearable. He develops obstructive symptoms in his bowels: bloating, abdominal pain, a lack of bowel output. Another colonoscopy is done, and a wire stent is inserted and inflated to relieve some of the blockage in his rectum.

The cancer accelerates. Tom dabbles in alternative therapies, which he pays for himself – terbinafine (an antifungal drug) and high-dose intravenous vitamin C. He tries statins (cholesterol-lowering medication), and metformin (a diabetes tablet) as advised by an alternative medicine specialist in London. Both Tom and his wife note that the vitamin C in particular is helpful, giving him more energy, enough even to get up and play with his children. 'When you live with a person with a terminal illness,' his wife tells me, 'it's the small things that matter the most.'

As Tom gets weaker, as his flesh melts down to his bones, as his freckles float unmoored on his concave cheeks, Jason does home visits to look after him while the local hospice provides oversight and support. Because of the Covid-19 pandemic, Jason has to don full PPE to visit. It is hot and sweaty under the mask and the gown but preventing infection in an immunocompromised patient is of paramount importance.

It is only in the last days of his life that Tom finally accepts his diagnosis. He asks Jason, 'Is this it, Doc? Is this the end?'

Jason looks at him frankly but kindly and says, 'Yes, Tom, I think it is.'

Tom and his wife cry and hug each other.

By this time, Jason has set up morphine drivers at home for Tom. Local district nurses help insert a nasogastric tube through Tom's nose to drain fluids from his stomach. Because Tom's gut has again obstructed from the rapid growth of tumour masses, fluid cannot drain away normally. He is now far too weak to tolerate any sort of surgical intervention.

Five days later, Tom dies at home. The medications that Jason has set up enable him to slip peacefully away. Tom's kids are on the bed beside him, holding onto their father's arms. Tom's wife and mother are by his side. Other whānau throng the room and sing songs of praise and sadness as he dies. It is a death that is as resonant with love, support and meaning as it can be.

***

Jason Tuhoe was born in Tūrangi, on the central North Island's volcanic plateau, surrounded by alpine desert and golden furry tussock. The landscape of his hometown was desolate, beautiful, chiselled by icy winds. Jason is the oldest in his family, and was brought up by his Māori mum and his Pākehā stepfather. Until he was ten years old, he believed that this man was his real dad, then he found out that his biological father was Māori. 'I suddenly didn't know who I was. I didn't know where I fitted in,' he says.

Jason started to act out. He nicked lollies from the village shop. He learnt to drive at the age of 12. He stole money left lying around the house and from his step-father's truck. It was rebellion against a man who now seemed to have no authentic authority over him. 'I was definitely headed down the prison track,' he says.

His mum packed him off to Hato Pāora College in Feilding, a boarding school for Māori students. He sees those years at Hato Pāora as invaluable: they straightened him out and gave him a sense of Māori identity and mana. He became the first in his family to finish high school, the first to go to university. He went to the University of Auckland's School of Medicine under the MAPAS programme (Māori and Pacific Admission Scheme). MAPAS helps counterbalance many of the systemic advantages that students from affluent families and suburbs hold over those from poorer areas. Over the course of many decades, this scheme has slowly built up numbers of Māori and Pasifika doctors to comprise 3.5 per cent and almost 2 per cent of the medical workforce respectively. This is still not properly representative of the population, which is 16 per cent Māori and 9 per cent Pasifika.

Jason met his medical wife during te reo Māori classes on campus. She has now completed a PhD in general surgery. While doing a run in general practice, Jason recognised its unique whanaungatanga. That sense of connection, of kinship, of relationship. And manaakitanga, caring for patients in as holistic a way as possible. These things resonated hugely. He worked with Dr James Te Whare, who looked after palliative-care patients in Ōtara, which piqued Jason's interest enough to complete a diploma in palliative medicine with the Totara Hospice in 2014.

Another important principle of palliative care resonated with Jason: tino rangatiratanga, self-determination, sovereignty. Palliative care, Jason believes, gives this to people. It gives them dignity, the right to live life till the end in the way they want to live it, despite insurmountable illness. It gives them the choice to determine where they will die, surrounded by loved ones, and to go home during the last days of their life, wherever home may be.

It's such a privilege to support a patient so that they can live well right until the end. Jason is used to the thanatophobia, the anxiety around death, a fear of dying, that envelops some patients struggling to accept their impending demise. He listens to the patient and walks alongside them rather than just offering advice and treatment.

**

'In this world nothing can be said to be certain, except death and taxes,' wrote Benjamin Franklin in 1789. Although death is an unalterable part of life, advances in medicine and science have depersonalised it, scrubbed it clean of resonance or meaning. Human perspectives on death have varied widely through history. In premodern times, it was common to die at a young age, from infectious diseases, poor sanitation, sabre-tooth tigers – a bumper crop of causes. Prior to curative surgery or chemotherapy, cancer was a fearful disease indeed. Weird lumps or pain or unusual symptoms ignited terror or a churlish insouciance. What recourse was there for something that was certain to kill you?

As longevity increased, death morphed into something to be at best ignored or, at worst, feared. The Welsh poet Dylan Thomas summed it up: 'Do not go gentle into that good night / Old age should burn and rave at close of day / Rage, rage, against the dying of the light.' This 'roistering, drunken and doomed poet' died aged just 39 of a combination of pneumonia and probable alcohol poisoning.

Attitudes towards death have been influenced by a reduction in religious beliefs, and a concomitant advance in pharmacological and other technological ways of managing death. Death can be delayed, but sometimes at the expense of quality of life. Death is further depersonalised by decisions being taken away from the person dying and their family members, and placed in the hands of medical personnel instead.

Science can articulate exactly what happens to the physical body after death, especially in cases where the expired flesh is not properly cared for, when people die alone and are not found for some time. There's rigor mortis, as limbs temporarily stiffen; bloating, as gut micro-organisms release toxic gases; skin slippage, as hydrolytic enzymes loosen the top layer of skin; and putrefaction. However, scientific knowledge and advances have not answered the unknown nature of life after death, if any such thing exists. There's also no quantifiable data that disproves the existence of an afterlife. Hence, people still fear death, the unknown and infinite nature of it. They may fear what happens after it, but also the process of death itself. Will it hurt like hell? What grief will it cause to loved ones?

The mention of 'palliative care' triggers a spectrum of responses. Some view it as if acceptance of their disease and the need for palliative care will legitimise their illness. Urban myths abound. There's a belief that palliative care is only available for people with cancer; that accepting palliative care means that the medics have 'given up'; that it serves to hasten death, often via the administration of morphine; and that it can only be provided in a clinical setting and not the patient's home.

The reality of palliative care, as Tom and his wife found, is far removed from these views. Distilled down to its essence, good palliative care allows a person with a life-limiting condition to live well so that they can die well. It is active and total care. Hospice care is a multimodal, comprehensive service that can assist a person at any age or stage who has a life-limiting illness – not just when nearing death. It focuses on the needs of the whole person, not just the treatment of their condition. It helps alleviate pain and suffering, identifies and treats physical, psychosocial and spiritual issues, and involves the wider family in a way that is holistic and inclusive. Good palliative care is invaluable in improving the quality of life for patients with life-threatening illness, and can be started a long time before death encroaches on life.

The modern palliative-care movement grew out of the hospice service, first set up by Dame Cicely Saunders in 1967. She opened St. Christopher's Hospice in London with an interdisciplinary team providing nursing, medical, social and religious care. Later, Professor Balfour Mount coined the term 'palliative care' when he brought the same service to Canada.

Good reading material on this topic includes *Being Mortal* by Dr Atul Gawande, an ultimately hopeful and powerful look at the ways that those who live well can die well. 'For human beings,' Gawande writes, 'life is meaningful because it is a story.' Another excellent book is *With the End in Mind: Dying, death and wisdom in an age of denial* by Dr Kathryn Mannix. This experienced palliative-care physician writes beautifully of the profound humanity of death. In her description of the process of death, she says, there is usually no flailing about, and rarely do the dying sit up in bed to give last words of wisdom. Dr Mannix describes it simply as 'our bodies running out of energy'.

She writes how, when someone is nearing death, they get tired, they sleep a lot. Mostly they'll be their normal selves while awake, but gradually, the amount of time they are asleep increases, until they become unconscious all the time. The automatic breathing reflex carries on, higher functions in the brain switch off. The muscles in the larynx might collapse a little, causing a sighing or groaning noise: a sign of unconsciousness, not distress. Breathing patterns alter, making it seem as if the dying person is gasping or struggling when, in fact, this is a reflex breathing pattern. They may make a rattling noise in their throat due to pooled secretions. Eventually, there will be a gentle breath out that is not followed by another breath in. Pain is not part of every death, but it can interrupt this sequence of events, and if so, good palliative care has strategies for managing this.

New Zealand's palliative-care service started in 1979 with the opening of Mary Potter Hospice in Wellington. It expanded with the founding of Hospice New Zealand in 1986. Currently, there are 33 hospice services nationally, and it is provided free of charge to residents and citizens. According to Hospice New Zealand, central government funding for their services is $155 million each year, while an additional $77 million needs to be fundraised annually. It is an important service that is still grossly underfunded. There are not enough palliative-care physicians for the population, and they are not equally accessible around New Zealand.

A palliative-care team includes physicians, nurses who do home visits to help with symptom management and can set up infusions of symptom-control medications, social workers, counsellors, dietitians, physiotherapists, and occupational therapists. As well as providing pain medication tailored to each patient's needs, the team offers support with managing personal cares. They'll give guidance on healthy eating, dealing with grief, networking with other support services and help with advanced-care planning, so that each patient can make informed decisions about how they want to live and die. There's support for caregivers, who are often under huge stress. There are bereavement groups for children, cultural and spiritual support, financial advice. It is, in every sense of the word, holistic.

In 2019, one in three people who died in New Zealand were supported by hospice. This amounted to 10,148 people. Many people under hospice care died at home (36 per cent, versus another 36 per cent in hospital and 26 per cent in aged residential care). However, 78 per cent were also cared for at home with no admission to an inpatient facility. People of all ages, and 130 different ethnic groups, used it. A quarter of hospice patients had a non-cancer diagnosis such as dementia, respiratory disease, motor neurone disease or multiple sclerosis.

In October 2020, New Zealanders voted to pass the End of Life Choice Act. The availability of euthanasia or assisted dying is something that many palliative-care physicians, and GPs with a special interest like Dr Tuhoe, have considered. There are safeguards around how patients will be able to access and utilise this Act. There are also areas of concern, for example, the lack of a sufficient 'cooling-off' period; no requirement to receive treatment first, or speak to a specialist; and no stipulation to have independent witnesses at any point during the process. The doctor providing the service need not have met the patient before, making it difficult to ascertain coercion. The art of prognostication – determining how long a person with a terminal illness has to live – is also remarkably inaccurate. Patients sometimes live for years when they've been given only a few months.

Ideally, New Zealand's already excellent palliative-care system, which provides so much comfort, grace and dignity to patients and their families, and does so in a medically ethical and holistic manner, would be expanded to meet the needs of all New Zealanders in their time of need.

***

The two years that Jason provided palliative care services to Tom are resonant with meaning. There were times of utter grief. There were times of despair and feeling defeated. But there were also glimpses of humanity stripped bare of the usual fetters of life. There were rich conversations, occasional laughter at absurdities, chances to say sorry and thank you and I love you.

For Tom's family, the fact that he was able to die in his own home, surrounded by his loved ones, remains a burnished and hallowed memory.

Jason feels honoured that he had the profound privilege of walking beside Tom in the last stages of his life. That he helped someone to live well until his last breath. And he has been reminded never to take his own health for granted.

Choosing the blue pill: when denial becomes deadly

patient: Carrie*; surgeon: Dr Lesina Nakhid-Schuster

Carrie* is a woman who presents to Auckland ED with concerning symptoms that she has had for months. It's clear that whatever she has is more than just the flu but, as Dr Lesina Nakhid-Schuster realises when she meets her, Carrie is in almost total denial about the severity of her symptoms. Carrie is in her fifties. She's a busy woman with lots to do and no time for sickness.

Denial seems to hold ransom the zeitgeist of our time, and not just in the medical sphere. Studies show that up to 80 per cent of the time, patients lie to their doctors about their diet, their exercise levels and their compliance with medications. Not that they deliberately lie – sometimes they don't notice or remember what they are eating. And sometimes the desire to impress their doctor is stronger than the drive to tell the truth.

Denial can also be a more absolute refutation of symptoms that are objectively concerning yet subjectively do not trigger alarm bells. As the author C. S. Lewis wrote, 'Denial is the shock absorber for the soul. It protects us until we are equipped to cope with reality.' It can provide a buffer against something that threatens to overwhelm us, it can allow us to inhabit a reality that is more soothing, less fretful, than the aggravating truth.

The 1999 film *The Matrix* depicts denial graphically. The protagonist, Neo, is offered the choice of a red pill or a blue pill by the enigmatic rebel leader Morpheus. The red pill represents reality but an uncertain future. The blue pill represents a beautiful prison: swallow it, Morpheus tells Neo, and you get to avoid real life, you get to stay in the simulated reality of the Matrix, where everything seems fine. Neo chooses the red pill, and thus chooses to find out 'how deep the rabbit hole goes'. Patient Carrie, meanwhile, appears to choose the blue pill: that is, the fragile 'prison' of imagined good health. Perhaps she suspects something is wrong but she is too frightened or too busy to allow medical reality to upend her life. So she carries on as if nothing is wrong, for months and months.

***

Lesina is in quarantine when I interview her. It is April 2020 and New Zealand is in the throes of a mellow autumn, overshadowed by the menace of pandemic. Newly returned from surgical registrar work in Australia, Lesina is at an Auckland hotel. She has plenty of time to do yoga. Occasionally someone knocks on the door, asks her a few basic health questions, points an infrared thermometer at her forehead, then moves on to the next quarantinee. The anodyne hotel room in which she is staying is in stark contrast to Auckland ED a decade earlier, where Lesina first met Carrie.

ED is busy that night. It is summer, and the air is sticky and a little humid in the maritime climate of New Zealand's largest city. Feet in soft shoes rush here and there. It's an intricate dance of doctors, nurses and orderlies in varying shades of blue. Endless cups of coffee are drunk to prop open tired eyes. Fluorescent lights flicker imperceptibly, bringing out the green in bruises, the sickly red of bloodied wounds. The smell of antiseptic swirls alongside tinctures of vomit and alcohol. Staff carry patient charts, tubes for intravenous fluids, medications. They wheel trolleys full of dressings and suturing equipment to cubicles. Rarely do they get time to sit and chat. It is only 11 pm, but the department is bursting at the seams.

Carrie has been brought into ED by her husband. She has been troubled by a persistent cough for the last two months. A smoker since her teens, she brushes this off as the proverbial 'smoker's cough', perhaps with a touch of infection on top. She is hopeful some antibiotics will knock it on its head. But her husband describes a shortness of breath that is not normal for

Carrie, even when just walking around their home in West Auckland, walking up the stairs, doing her normal chores. She's lost weight without intending to, and has started cutting back on her activities.

Both Carrie and her husband strike Lesina as salt-of-the-earth sorts. They come from farming stock and have a 'get on with it' mentality. They've lived in West Auckland for several decades, which is a point of connection for Lesina: she's also a 'Westie', even if she eschews the calcified artery that is Lincoln Road, with all its greasy fast-food joints, for the fresh air of the mountains and the wildness of the west coast beaches.

Unfortunately for Carrie, she is also a chronic avoider of medical establishments. The doctor, Carrie believes, is an incidental extra to her busy life, to be consulted only when in dire straits. If you lead an active life, she tells Lesina, and if you are reasonably healthy with just one or two vices, then you don't need to see a doctor regularly. Who knows, you may just get by with good genes and a smidgen of luck.

There are historical examples that might support what medics could regard as a somewhat cavalier approach to life. Take Jeanne Calment. This Frenchwoman from Arles was the oldest-known person recorded, and lived to be 122 years old, despite smoking for 100 of these years. A century of cigarettes! Unless you have inherited her genetic fortitude, however, her recipe for longevity is not to be recommended.

'The thing that stood out for me was how Carrie thought her health was pretty much okay,' says Lesina, a house officer (junior doctor) at the time. 'Carrie was in her late fifties. She was a long-term smoker and hadn't been to the doctors for 20 years. Not one single time, she claimed. Didn't have a regular GP. Hadn't done any routine checks like a mammogram or a smear, etc. Her husband practically forced her to hospital because her cough had become so bad.'

Carrie has lines around her lips and eyes, and dull, dry skin – the legacy of decades of nicotine and carbon monoxide suffocating her blood flow and displacing sweet fresh oxygen. She is reasonably chirpy and upbeat, telling Lesina, 'I don't even know why I'm here. I feel silly. You must be so busy. I'm just wasting everyone's time. Just need a quick check-up then I can be on my way.'

During the initial assessment, Carrie's blood pressure and pulse are normal. She has a low-grade temperature and her oxygen saturations are lowish, sitting at 92 per cent. Her cough is hacking and painful to hear. She is clearly dyspnoeic (short of breath), even at rest. Lesina listens to her chest, palpates her abdomen, orders blood tests and a chest X-ray. The radiograph shows numerous patchy 2–3-millimetre opacities throughout both of Carrie's lungs. To a layperson, this would look like a ghostly white tree branching in all directions, with multiple little nubbins on the branches. Strange fruit, of no good origin.

'This is unusual,' the senior says to Lesina. 'You should talk to radiology about this.'

It is 2 am by now. The cardinal rule of junior doctorhood is not to disturb senior colleagues for non-urgent matters; waking a sleeping radiologist for something as relatively minor as a chest X-ray transgresses medical etiquette, so Lesina decides the radiologist should be rung in the morning. She starts Carrie on antibiotics for presumed pneumonia and admits her to a general medical ward for further work-up. 'The differential diagnosis included atypical pneumonia, tuberculosis, sarcoidosis, fungal infections, occupational lung disease and metastatic cancer.' As Carrie is a long-term smoker, the dreaded C-word lurks.

Before Carrie is wheeled up to the ward, her husband kisses her goodnight, promising to return a few hours later for the morning round. 'Carrie looked pretty unconcerned,' remembers Lesina. 'Just matter-of-fact, calm. She was not prepared to entertain the possibility of serious disease. She thought she felt reasonably well and would have gone home with tablets if she could.'

Lesina finishes her ED placement a few days later and starts work as a house officer in a general medicine run. Two weeks after she first met Carrie, she is called to certify a patient's death on one of the wards. This will be her first death certificate.

Medical students are exposed to death during their training, usually in the form of specimens floating in formalin. An amputated leg, scabbed with hard black eschar, the end result of someone's poorly controlled diabetes. A heart, sliced open to reveal the thumb-sized clot that undid that engine of life. A cross-section of emphysematous lung, coarsely honeycombed. Doing that first death certificate, however, is always somewhat nerve-racking. If the room is empty except for the medic and the body, it is all too easy to imagine a phantom heart beating when one auscultates the chest, or to imagine the slow rise and fall of stiff cold ribs.

'As soon as I walked into the room, I recognised Carrie's husband. The room was full of relatives. Then I saw Carrie, lying on the bed. I was shocked,' Lesina recalls. 'The husband started crying when he saw me. I could not believe that someone who had been walking around just two weeks previously could have gone downhill so fast.'

Lesina is unable to stop crying. 'Truly, I was legit sobbing.' She cries so hard that a nurse suggests she leave the room and come back when she is more composed. This nurse is a seasoned ward warrior; Lesina is well down the pecking order and is showing unreasonable amounts of emotion. As medical students, the importance of 'empathy with boundaries' is drummed in during lectures – the ability to separate our own emotions from those of the patient is a skill learnt over years and years, and it is an imperfect skill.

Carrie's notes show she's had a battery of tests since Lesina saw her. Carrie was tested for infection, as her initial X-ray looked similar to that of patients with pneumonia (in particular, community-acquired atypical pneumonia). She was cleared of tuberculosis, HIV or fungus as being the culprits. She was checked for hypersensitivity pneumonitis. Then a CT scan of her chest confirmed miliary disease – millet-like 2–3-millimetre infiltrates in both lungs, as well as enlarged lymph nodes in her mediastinum. Further CT scans of her abdomen and pelvis showed enlarged nodes in these areas. But the brain scan was clear.

A bronchoscopy, bronchoalveolar lavage and fluoroscopy-guided transbronchial biopsies were performed, where a camera was inserted into the lungs and samples collected. This was done while Carrie was still relatively stable and able to tolerate the procedure. The diagnosis was obtained via the biopsies: primary adenocarcinoma of the lung, with spread through the lymphatic system to give lymphangitis carcinomatosa.

Our lymphatic system is a network of vessels throughout our bodies. It carries lymph fluid (which is composed partly of absorbed fats from our gut, infection-fighting cells and cell debris) upwards and eventually back into the blood stream. Lymph nodes are security stations along the way that trap pathogens and cancer cells in an attempt to prevent spread. The lymphatic spread of cancer cells is what causes the miliary tree-like pattern on imaging. A malignant miliary pattern on the lungs is more often due to breast, thyroid or renal cancers that have spread via the blood and seeded into the lungs, rather than arising primarily from the lungs. Primary adenocarcinomas of the lung that show a miliary pattern have a poor prognosis and don't respond well to treatment.

Lesina returns to the room once she has composed herself, certifies the death and fills out the death certificate. The family decline an autopsy, but it is assumed that Carrie's sudden death is due to a massive pulmonary embolus – a large, wobbly blood clot in the lungs, a known sequelae of malignancy, and one that can cause cardiac arrest.

***

Lung cancer is the leading cause of cancer death in New Zealand, in large part because, by the time it is discovered, it has already spread and is difficult to treat. Hence the five-year survival rate is only 17 per cent; many patients are already at stage IV of the disease when they are diagnosed. The most common subset (80–85 per cent) of lung cancers is non-small-cell lung cancer, with adenocarcinomas the most common sort in this group. The other subset is made up of small-cell lung cancers.

Lung cancer is of course strongly linked to smoking, aberrations such as the long-lived Frenchwoman Jeanne Calment notwithstanding. Tobacco smoke contains some 4000 different chemicals, many of which are carcinogenic (cancer-causing). These chemicals damage our DNA repeatedly and with wild abandon. Smoking not only causes lung cancer, but also cancers of the mouth, throat, oesophagus, larynx, and further afield to create sinister mayhem in the pancreas, bladder and bowels. Smoking doesn't just stop at the big C; it also leads to heart disease and other forms of lung disease, and prevents our skin and bones from healing quickly after injury.

There is a protracted push by public health authorities to discourage smoking. Currently 87.5 per cent of New Zealanders are smoke-free. The aim is for 100 per cent by the year 2025 – aided by exorbitant taxes and gruesome photos on the sides of the packets.

The latest statistics show a stark difference between Māori and non-Māori rates of smoking. While overall adult rates have dropped to 12.5 per cent, they remain high in Māori men (31.5 per cent) and even higher in Māori women (36 per cent). The smoking rate for Pasifika adults is 24 per cent. Given that these ethnic groups have higher rates of death and tobacco-related illness, it is imperative to target tobacco-reduction measures to these communities as much as possible. Perhaps 10–15 per cent of those who develop lung cancer may have never smoked. Passive smoking can increase the risk of developing lung cancer by up to 30 per cent. Conversely, not everyone who smokes goes on to develop lung cancer, indicating that there is a complex interplay between genetic factors and carcinogens.

Carrie's trajectory from reasonably independent life to death is so short that, to this day, Lesina wonders if being given the diagnosis somehow punctured Carrie's buoyant sense of self-sufficiency. Did she simply give up? Did denial offer her a modicum of protection?

***

Lesina was born near the Mississippi, in the sweltering heat of New Orleans. The multicultural make-up of her birthplace is reflected in her own ancestry. Lesina's mother is a second-generation Trinidadian, with one Lebanese parent; her father is a New Zealander of Samoan and German ancestry. They met in Trinidad, and were en route to New Zealand, via the States, when Lesina was born.

Lesina's mother is an associate professor at Auckland University of Technology, and researches Māori and Pasifika educational achievement and culturally relevant research methodologies. 'My mum is proud of being black, and is an activist through and through,' Lesina says. 'I usually prefer to blend in more!' Her father was a geography teacher at Mt Albert Grammar School, but is now retired.

An early influence and role model in Lesina's life was Richard Douglas, an ear, nose and throat surgeon. 'He was so dedicated to helping people. Mum also brought around awesome Māori and Pacific Island women doctors to talk to me when I was considering med school,' says Lesina. 'That was really influential and inspiring, to be able to see people who looked like me being doctors.' However, she said she found the subjects that are a prerequisite for medical school a hard slog. 'I had to do the basic sciences with gritted teeth. Until then, I had been doing a lot of drama and arts subjects, which I absolutely loved.'

At the School of Medicine at the University of Auckland, Lesina felt the weight of being a minority. Her classmates were generally from posher central suburbs. There was also a peculiar type of prejudice that those of mixed race grapple with: off-hand comments such as 'you're not that brown' or 'you don't act like those Pasifika' felt like veiled insults. 'On the whole, though, I didn't really have heaps of racism thrown at me. Perhaps it's like what Meghan Markle says – if you look a little bit racially ambiguous, you can fit in anywhere.' Once she graduated, she took a year out in 2015 to study acting. After some commercial work in Australia, Lesina became New Zealand's first *Bachelorette*. However, she was taken aback at the tumult of negative feedback on social media. 'Pure racism. So much online chatter about how I wasn't a "real" New Zealander, even though I've lived here my whole life. Lily [McManus, the other bachelorette who was brought in part way through the show] didn't get one jot of that – ironically, she's Australian!'

Lesina went to Australia in 2019 to escape the treadmill that is the New Zealand medical system. 'In New Zealand, there is so much pressure to succeed. It's also quite gossipy; everyone knows everyone else. Australia is so much bigger, more anonymous, and it is more acceptable to pursue a wide variety of career paths, rather than aiming in a straight line for a consultant's position from day one. You can be a private surgical assistant long-term in Aussie – more of a middle person, but with plenty of great hands-on work and the added bonus of flexibility to pursue other interests. It totally takes away that anxiety of having to achieve, of having to get to the top.'

The work she enjoys most now is fixing things up to make them look better. She has worked as a surgical registrar in plastics, in ear, nose and throat, and in general surgical disciplines. 'Surgery feels almost like sculpting. It is creative in many ways, as much as acting or painting.'

She says that junior doctors get thrown into the deep end a lot more in New Zealand. 'That can be both a good and a bad thing. On one hand, you learn a lot, and you learn it quickly.' Junior doctors in South Africa are treated with even greater abandon, forced as they are to do caesarean sections on women in rural areas with very little training.

'In Australia things are much more privatised and consultant-led, so there is that assurance of having really good oversight. There is also much more of a focus on money in Oz, which I think unfortunately can affect how you do your work; your altruism, for example, can get suffocated by the relentless focus on adequate compensation. People are scrupulous about charging overtime, whereas in New Zealand it is just in our culture to work overtime and not always charge for it. It's more of a get on with it, non-complaining culture.'

Lesina intends to head back to Australia, to continue to practice the sort of medicine she loves while also trying to establish a creative career.

**

Truth be told, it is likely that Carrie had a poor prognosis when she presented to ED. If she'd perhaps had a regular doctor, had gone for regular check-ups, had quit smoking years earlier, perhaps such things might have prevented her untimely death. But it is fascinating to look at how our minds influence our bodies, whether through intentional focused attention, through denial or at least a desire to not wallow in 'what if' outcomes but maintain a relatively positive mind-set.

The Shaolin monks of China take intentional focused attention to another level. They perform physical feats that should be painful to them but are not, such as tying heavy iron rollers to their testicles and dragging them around. The monks manage to block out pain by practising Qigong, a meditation that integrates physical postures, breathing techniques and focused intention. Another example of focused attention is Wim Hof, a Dutch extreme athlete known as The Iceman who has set world records for swimming the longest distance under ice, and has run the fastest barefoot half-marathon on ice and snow. Wearing only shorts and no shoes, he has climbed to the summits of Mt Everest and Mt Kilimanjaro. He credits his endurance to breathing techniques and meditation.

Clearly we can train our minds to alter our perception of pain, but the role of denial in patients who have been given life-altering diagnoses is complex. Often, society views denial in disparaging terms. Man (or woman) up, we say. Face up to your issues, own them, overcome them. Whether it is smoking or alcohol or chocolate biscuits.

Medical professionals are frequently frustrated or saddened by patients who stubbornly refute objective evidence of their own morbidity. The onset of illness triggers psychological distress, which can then trigger defence mechanisms as we scramble to cope. Unlike other coping strategies, denial as a defence is often unintentional and comes into play to reduce anxiety. Short-term denial can be helpful. It helps us deal with medical situations where we've suddenly lost control. However, longer-term denial can be maladaptive and can cause serious psychological disturbance.

Initial research into denial in the 1950s and 1960s looked into its role only in neurological or psychiatric conditions, rather than somatic (bodily) diseases. In the 1970s, researchers started to investigate the role of denial in cardiac and oncological settings. Denial is hard to objectively identify and quantify: it is part of the shifting sands of response to and coping with illness. A patient may be in denial of their diagnosis, in denial of the impact of the diagnosis on their lifestyle (and hence be resistant to change), or in denial of the negative emotions associated with the diagnosis. Or a combination of all these elements.

Despite moves to make medical care more patient-centred, there is still a tendency from medics to pathologise non-compliant patient behaviour. And the experience of someone else's denial can be subjective. What could seem like denial to one health professional may be perceived as an appropriate coping strategy by another. Medics can mislabel a person's behaviour as denial when it might be more accurately characterised as optimism.

Studies have shown, oddly, that partial denial of a cancer diagnosis, or at least denial of the awfulness of treatment, can have beneficial effects. A study of breast-cancer patients showed that patients who held negative or highly negative expectations about the side effects of treatment experienced almost twice the side effects of those with positive or low negative expectations.[29] In other words, reality bites. And a 2009 thesis concludes: 'Lung cancer patients displaying greater denial reported a better overall perception of health and better physical functioning. They also suffered less from dyspnea, fatigue, gastrointestinal symptoms, dysphagia and arm pain. Thus, denial may be adaptive in lung cancer patients … Our main and most interesting finding is that patients fare better when they express a moderate level of denial or increase their level of denial over time. Patients showing little denial proved to experience worse social and emotional outcomes, and overall quality of life.'[30]

Denial of disease is complex. It can fluctuate in intensity during an illness. Clearly in some instances it leads to poor, potentially preventable outcomes, as it did in Carrie's case. All these years later, Carrie's case remains a vivid example to Lesina of how someone in denial can simply, stubbornly, push on through, for a lot longer than they might otherwise have done. Denial in patients can be frustrating for medical professionals, who are taught to inform patients of illness and who expect patients to acknowledge this so that holistic care can be provided. But far from being simply an irrational and obstructive response, perhaps denial is also a form of hope. Perhaps it allows some patients to persevere in the face of incredible odds, at least for some time.

Acknowledgements

It's been something of a communal effort, this book, and my grateful thanks and appreciation go to the following people:

To Steve Braunias for kickstarting it by asking me to write two essays for *Newsroom* – huzzah! And to publisher Alex Hedley, for graciously taking a chance on a literary nobody.

Thanks to all the interviewees who so generously gave of their time, memories, stories and knowledge to help me craft this book.

Then, in no particular order, to the medical colleagues, experts and friendly writers who provided me with valuable information and feedback. Firstly, the medics, many of whom are friends: doctors Samantha Murton, Vinod Singh, Heidi Conway and Katrina Kirikino-Cox (general practitioner specialists), Dr David Galler (intensive care specialist), Dr Jith Somaratne (cardiologist), Dr Derek Luo (gastroenterologist), doctors Libby

King and Suzanne Poole (respiratory physicians), Dr Renee Liang (paediatrician), Dr Louise Tomlinson (obstetrician), Mrs Jenny Wagener and Mr James McKay (surgeons), Dr Damian Tomic (chief medical advisor, Department of Corrections).

The fantastic writers and friends: Dame Fiona Kidman, Vincent O'Malley, Joshua Teal, David Honiss, Gail Oats, Anne Humphries (also a nurse), David Robinson.

And the experts: Te Miringa Tahana Waipouri-Voykovic (Kaumātua), Professor Tracey McIntosh (Indigenous Studies, University of Auckland), Dr Dean Vuksanovic (senior psychologist, Gold Coast Hospital), Rebecca Powell (Comms, Department of Corrections), Lisa Meadows (PRIME), Linda Reynolds (NZ Rural GP Network).

Lastly, a huge thank you to my lovely husband, Ian, and to my delicious parents, Ranjit and Sirina, for always being so proud and encouraging of my writing. Love you!

Endnotes

PART 1: Sudden events
One bullet, one man

1   Patricia E McDonald et al, 'The effect of acceptance training on psychological and physical health outcomes in elders with chronic conditions', *Journal of the National Black Nurses Association*, Vol 22, December 2011; Ramony Chan, 'The effect of acceptance on health outcomes in patients with chronic kidney disease', *Nephrology Dialysis Transplant*, Vol 28, 2013; and Devika Duggal, Amanda Sacks-Zimmerman and Taylor Liberta, 'The impact of hope and resilience on multiple factors in neurosurgical patients', *Cureus*, Vol 8, October 2016.

2   Y Nestoriuc et al, 'Is it best to expect the worst? Influence of patients' side-effect expectations on endocrine treatment outcome in a 2-year prospective clinical cohort study', *Annals of Oncology*, Vol 27, 2016.

Hongi the wairua

3   Adam Fogel et al, 'Cultural Assessment and Treatment of Psychiatric Patients'; ncbi.nlm.nih.gov/books/NBK482311, published online.

4   Patte Randal and Nick Argyle, 'Spiritual emergency – a useful explanatory model?' in Spirituality SIG publications, 2006.

5   According to the late Reverend Māori Marsden.

PART 2: The things we carry

A midnight epiphany on childhood

6   Seth D Pollak et al, 'Differences in brain structure development may explain test score gap for poor children', *JAMA Network Journals*, 20 July 2015.

7   American Psychological Association, *Education and Socioeconomic Status Factsheet*, July 2017, and 'Family income, parental education and brain structure in children and adolescents', *Nature Neuroscience* Vol 18, 2015.

8   'Understanding the Effects of Maltreatment on Brain Development', April 2015, www.childwelfare.gov/pubPDFs/brain_development.pdf

9   Johnna R Swartz, Ahmad R Hariri and Douglas E Williamson, 'An epigenetic mechanism links socioeconomic status to changes in depression-related brain function in high-risk adolescents', *Molecular Psychiatry*, 24 May 2016.

10   Kimberly G Noble et al, 'Family income, parental education and brain structure in children and adolescents', *Nature Neuroscience*, Vol 18, 2015. See also Colter Mitchell et al, 'Social disadvantage, genetic sensitivity, and children's telomere length', PNAS, 111(16), April 2014.

11   Kathryn Wilson, David J Hansen and Ming Li, 'The traumatic stress response in child maltreatment and resultant neuropsychological effects', *Aggression and Violent Behaviour*, 16(2), 2011.

The greatness and pain that our ancestors gave

12   A Waitangi Tribunal inquiry ('The economic rehabilitation of Māori veterans', May 2018) tallies 4995 Māori ex-service people after WWII. The report states: 'The actual number settled with rehabilitation assistance appears to have been 217, 27 years after the end of World War II.' Two hundred and seventeen out of 4995 Māori ex-service men and women is 4.3 per cent. By contrast, 12,249 of all other veterans, out of a total of 197,270, were settled on the land with rehabilitation assistance (6.21 per cent).The rates of post-war settlement were also much slower for Māori, partly due to

incorrect assumptions about land ownership, and multiple agencies handling rehabilitation assistance. The rates of educational loans for ex-soldiers were lower for Māori, 3 per cent versus 10.7 per cent for Pākehā. When it came to housing loans, Māori fared better, with proportionately more housing loans (36 per cent versus 34 per cent), of higher value (£1900 versus £1600). This was likely in recognition of the dire state of pre-war Māori housing and living standards. However, Māori were given business loans less often (4.8 per cent versus 5.8 per cent) and the loans were of significantly lower value than those given to non-Māori (£440 versus £534). Resettlement on farms was lower for Māori (4.6 per cent versus 6.2 per cent), and a process of 'tagging' meant that Māori were often unable to ballot for prime, productive Crown land.

13 A report in 2019 by the Health Quality and Safety Commission ('A window on the quality of Aotearoa New Zealand's Health Care') is damning. Māori women have poorer access to maternity care, with more babies who are small for gestational age. Māori children have poorer access to dental care, especially in rural areas. Like Pasifika people, Māori are less likely to be referred to specialist care, and then wait longer to see the specialist (at least in the under-65 group). In those over 65, Māori are more likely to be prescribed combinations of medications that can cause kidney failure. Māori with disabilities are less likely to be supplied with the specialist equipment they need. Māori children have higher rates of asthma-reliever medicine prescribed with no preventer, possibly contributing to 30 per cent higher hospitalisation rates. Suicide rates are higher in young Māori. Acute hospital admission rates are higher, including for preventable illnesses. Māori die from treatable diseases at rates that are two and a half times that of non-Māori. There are much higher rates of certain cancers in Māori, such as lung and stomach cancer, linked partly to increased rates of smoking and infection. Māori with diabetes are less likely to receive good monitoring. Māori are more likely to report barriers such as cost in accessing healthcare, and to report poorer experiences of hospital-level care.

Meth, manslaughter and mercy

14   For example, for the same crime, 18 per cent of Māori will receive a prison sentence, versus 11 per cent of Pākehā (Statistics NZ and the Department of Corrections). The crimes range from petty theft to burglary to homicide to sexual assault, but the same trend is seen in each category – much higher incarceration rates for Māori. Even for low-level crimes such as drug use or possession, 2 per cent of Pākehā who are convicted go to prison, versus 7.3 per cent of Māori. The incarceration figures for Māori wāhine, meanwhile, are literally criminal. Māori women are the most heavily incarcerated indigenous group in the world, making up 63 per cent of New Zealand's female prisoners. This is despite Māori making up just 16.5 per cent of the population. It's a shameful statistic to be known for as a nation.

15   Ninety-one per cent of prisoners surveyed had a lifetime diagnosis of a mental-health or substance-abuse disorder. Sixty-two per cent had either a mental-health or a substance-use disorder in the 12 months prior; 20 per cent had both (substance misuse in the general population is 32 per cent; Ministry of Health, 2017). Seven per cent had psychotic symptoms – hearing voices that were not there, seeing things that no one else could see. A quarter of respondents had depression (versus 20 per cent for the general population). Another quarter met the criteria for an anxiety disorder, such as PTSD or stress (compared with 19 per cent of the general population). Overall, 62 per cent had a 12-month incidence of any mental-health disorder, which was thrice that of the general population incidence of 21 per cent. Six per cent had attempted suicide. Less than half of those surveyed with mental-health or substance-use disorders had received any form of medical or psychological treatment. The data is worse for female prisoners: 52 per cent of women in prison have a lifetime incidence of PTSD, 75 per cent of women in prison have diagnosed mental-health problems (versus 61 per cent of male prisoners), 46 per cent have a lifetime alcohol dependence (versus 35 per cent for the men), 68 per cent have been the victim of family violence, 44 per cent have drug-dependence disorders (versus 37 per cent of male prisoners).

16   T Mitchell, A Theadom and E Du Preez, 'Prevalence of Traumatic
      Brain Injury in a Male Adult Prison Population and Links With
      Offence Type', Neuroepidemiology (2017) Vol 48. Mitchell et al found
      that 63.8 per cent of New Zealand male offenders had sustained a TBI
      across their lifetime; 32.5 per cent had experienced multiple injuries.
      A paper by Schofield et al in 2015 showed that sustaining a TBI in
      childhood increased one's chances of imprisonment in adulthood.
      This indicates that, for some, a TBI precedes offending. Other studies
      have found that those with TBI have higher rates of violent offending,
      especially sexual offending, younger age of offending, and higher rates
      of reoffending. People with TBIs are more likely to be unemployed,
      and more likely to engage in antisocial behaviour.

17   The UK's Dyslexia Institute estimates dyslexia prevalence in prisoners
      is three to four times that of the general population. A study of
      Texan prisoners found that 48 per cent of the sample was dyslexic
      (Moody et al, 2000). Other studies in the UK have found a 30 to
      45 per cent incidence of attention deficit hyperactivity disorder in
      youth prisoners. This is at least a five-fold increase compared to
      non-prisoners. For adults, the rates were up to 30 per cent, at least a
      ten-fold increase. Rates of autism spectrum disorders in maximum
      security prisoners in the US were also four-fold that of the general
      population (Fazio, Pietz and Denney, 2012).

A grumpy man

18   The life expectancy for Pasifika New Zealanders hovers at five years
      less than the New Zealand average (Statistics NZ). The median net
      worth (assets minus liabilities) of an average Pasifika New Zealander
      is just $15,000 in 2018 figures. The median wealth of a Pākehā is
      $138,000. For Asians, net worth is $46,000; for Māori, $28,000.
      Pasifika are the least likely ethnic group to own their own home
      (less than 20 per cent do, and the numbers are dropping). Around
      one in ten New Zealanders live in crowded homes; for Pasifika, that
      figure is four in ten. About one-third of Pasifika children live in poor
      households. According to the 2018 census, two out of five Māori

and Pasifika in private dwellings live in damp conditions, with a concomitant increase in communicable diseases, respiratory illness and rheumatic fever.

Cardiovascular disease is the principle cause of death for Pasifika peoples (Ministry of Health). Death rates from stroke are higher than for other ethnic groups. Disparities in cancer survival have unfortunately increased in the last 25 years. Lung cancer and liver cancer rates are higher in Pasifika men than in the general population; breast and cervical cancer rates are higher in Pasifika women. Mental-health disease rates are higher than the general population, yet access to mental-health services is very low. Access to screening measures and specialist care is lower, leading to avoidable mortality.

Two-thirds of Pasifika New Zealand adults are obese, one-third of Pasifika children are also. This is linked to less physical activity and poorer diets. This then segues into higher rates of diabetes, with Pasifika adults having 2.8 times the diabetes rate of non-Pasifika New Zealanders. Despite high attendance, Pasifika people still have poorer outcomes and are less often referred to specialists, despite their higher burden of disease. Pasifika peoples with disabilities are less likely to receive help than their non-Pasifika peers.

Pasifika children have the highest hospitalisation rates for acute and chronic respiratory and infectious diseases of any group in New Zealand. This includes diseases such as rheumatic fever, traditionally a disease of poorer countries. It also includes bronchiectasis, dental disease, gastroenteritis and kidney infections. Chronic illness in childhood has knock-on effects in later life.

PART 3: Time proves everything
A fat bomb a day keeps the doctor away

19   Carol F Kirkpatrick et al, 'Review of current evidence and clinical recommendations on the effects of low-carbohydrate and very-low-carbohydrate (including ketogenic) diets for the management of body

weight and other cardiometabolic risk factors', *Journal of Clinical Lipidology*, 13(5), 1 September 1 2019.

20   Shaminie J Athinarayanan et al, 'Long-term effects of a novel, continuous, remote-care intervention including nutritional ketosis for the management of Type 2 diabetes: A 2-year non-randomised clinical trial', *Frontiers in Endocrinology*, 5 June 2019.

21   Matthew CL Phillips et al, 'Low-fat versus ketogenic diet in Parkinson's disease: A pilot randomised controlled trial', *Movement Disorders*, 11 August 2018.

22   Phillips et al, hypothesised that two years of fasting and ketogenic diet therapy weakened the malignant cells in the thymoma. This potentially 'set the stage'. It was only when Sarona had two serious relapses of her myasthenia, associated with activated immune function, loss of appetite and weight loss (11 per cent of body weight, then 28 per cent of body weight), that significant reductions in the tumour size occurred (32 per cent decrease in size during the first relapse, 96 per cent decrease in size during the second relapse). Perhaps immune activation and extreme energy restriction contributed to the regressions. Perhaps 'spontaneous regression', which has been documented multiple times in many cancers, occurred as a sequelae of this immune activation (however, spontaneous regression of metastatic thymoma is extremely rare). It is also possible that the prednisone that was used in the second relapse also led to the death of lymphocytes (immune cells that make up thymomas alongside cancer cells), further enhancing regression.

    The most plausible hypothesis, the researchers conclude, is that 'two years of fasting and ketogenic diet therapy metabolically weakened the thymoma, setting the stage for a combined immunity-induced, metabolic-induced, and prednisone-induced near-complete regression.' Matthew CL Phillips et al, 'Managing Metastatic Thymoma with Metabolic and Medical Therapy: a case report', *Frontiers in Oncology*, 5 May 2020.

That silence where no sound may be

23   Rachel Simon-Kumar, 'Ethnic perspectives on family violence in Aotearoa, New Zealand', *New Zealand Family Violence Clearinghouse*, Issues Paper 14, April 2019.

The changing face of general practice

24   Wilfred Owen, 'Anthem for Doomed Youth', 1917.

25   Zara Mason, Chrys Jaye and Dawn Miller, 'General Practitioners providing obstetric care in New Zealand. What differentiates GPs who continue to deliver babies?' *Journal of Primary Health Care*, 9(1), 2017.

26   David M Levine, Bruce E Landon and Jeffrey A Linder, 'Quality and experience of outpatient care in the United States for adults with or without primary care', *Journal of the American Medical Association*, 179(3), January 2019, 363–372.

Going home

27   Katrina J Sharples et al, 'The New Zealand PIPER Project: colorectal cancer survival according to rurality, ethnicity and socioeconomic deprivation – results from a retrospective cohort study', *New Zealand Medical Journal*, Vol 131, 2018.

28   Marzieh Araghi et al, 'Changes in colorectal cancer incidence in seven high income countries: a population-based study', *The Lancet*, 4(7), 1 July 2019.

Choosing the blue pill: when denial becomes deadly

29   Y Nestoriuc et al, 'Is it best to expect the worst? Influence of patients' side-effect expectations on endocrine treatment outcome in a 2-year prospective clinical cohort study', *Annals of Oncology*, Vol 27, 2016.

30   Tineke Vos, *Denial and Quality of Life in Lung Cancer Patients*, University of Amsterdam, 2009.